Handbook of Practical Pharmacology - I

Authored by

Suman Kamlesh Rattan
Department of Pharmacy
A Central University,
Guru Ghasidas Vishwavidyalaya
Bilaspur, Chhattisgarh 495009, India

Kedar Prasad Meena
Department of Pharmacy,
A Central University,
Guru Ghasidas Vishwavidyalaya
Bilaspur, Chhattisgarh 495009, India

&

Venu Anand Das Vaishnav
Department of Pharmacy (Neuropharmacology)
A Central University,
Guru Ghasidas Vishwavidyalaya
Bilaspur, Chhattisgarh 495009, India

Handbook of Practical Pharmacology - I

Authors: Suman Kamlesh Rattan, Kedar Prasad Meena and Venu Anand Das Vaishnav

ISBN (Online): 979-8-89881-219-5

ISBN (Print): 979-8-89881-220-1

ISBN (Paperback): 979-8-89881-221-8

Published by Bentham Science Publishers Pte. Ltd. Singapore,

in collaboration with Eureka Conferences, USA. All Rights Reserved.

First published in 2025.

need for a court order if at any point you breach any terms of this License Agreement. In no event will any delay or failure by Bentham Science Publishers in enforcing your compliance with this License Agreement constitute a waiver of any of its rights.

3. You acknowledge that you have read this License Agreement, and agree to be bound by its terms and conditions. To the extent that any other terms and conditions presented on any website of Bentham Science Publishers conflict with, or are inconsistent with, the terms and conditions set out in this License Agreement, you acknowledge that the terms and conditions set out in this License Agreement shall prevail.

Bentham Science Publishers Pte. Ltd.
No. 9 Raffles Place
Office No. 26-01
Singapore 048619
Singapore
Email: subscriptions@benthamscience.net

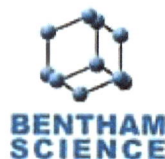

CONTENTS

FOREWORD

Pharmacology is the bedrock of effective clinical practice, translating the science of drugs into tangible patient outcomes. In this rapidly advancing field, access to clear, useful, and application-focused information that improve the comprehension of drug actions, interactions, and therapeutic applications is becoming more and more crucial.

The *"Handbook of Practical Pharmacology - I"* is a comprehensive and practical resource designed for the modern learners including students, teachers, and medical professionals. This book offers a methodical and practical approach to pharmacological concepts, complete with key drug profiles, well-structured experiments, and crucial insights into pharmacodynamic and pharmacokinetic ideas. Through the integration of theoretical knowledge and practical applications, this handbook enables students to understand basic pharmacological procedures and their practical applications.

This handbook's clarity, accuracy, and dedication to promoting a deeper comprehension of pharmacology beyond rote memorizing are what make it especially important. For the upcoming generation of healthcare workers, it fosters critical thinking, problem-solving, and evidence-based decision-making skills that are essential.

The authors have done a commendable task by producing a resource that will surely help students grasp the intricacies of pharmacology. I have no doubt that this handbook will be a trustworthy ally on the academic path of future pharmacologists and practitioners, providing them the essential knowledge and practical skills, they need to navigate the complexities of pharmacology with confidence and competence.

Preeti K. Suresh
University Institute of Pharmacy
Pt. Ravishankar Shukla University
Raipur, Chhattisgarh, India

PREFACE

With great pleasure, we present the "Handbook of Practical Pharmacology - I," which is devoted to the teachers and students of this nation's pharmacy institutes. This book was created and edited in compliance with the Pharmacy Council of India's (PCI) "Practical Pharmacology-I" syllabus requirement for the second year (4th semester) B. Pharm. degree in pharmacy, as stated in the "Bachelor of Pharmacy (B. Pharm.) course regulations 2014." The book is broken up into fifteen chapters, which are as follows:

Chapter 1: Introduction to experimental pharmacology

Chapter 2: Instruments used in the experimental pharmacology laboratory

Chapter 3: Study of common laboratory animals

Chapter 4: Maintenance of laboratory animals as per CCSEA guidelines

Chapter 5: Commonly used laboratory techniques

Chapter 6: Study of different routes of drug administration in murines

Chapter 7: Effects of hepatic microsomal enzyme inducers on phenobarbitone-induced sleep duration in mice

Chapter 8: Drugs acting on ciliary motility of frog oesophagus

Chapter 9: Impact of several drugs on the rabbit eye

Chapter 10: Impact of skeletal muscle relaxants assessed *via* Rotarod apparatus

Chapter 11: Effect of drugs on locomotor activity of mice using Actophotometer

Chapter 12: Anticonvulsant effect of drugs by the MES and PTZ method

Chapter 13: Drugs used for anti-cationic activity and stereotype-like behavior in murines

Chapter 14: Study of anxiolytic activity of drugs using mice/rats

Chapter 15: Study of local anaesthetics by different methods

CCSEA Guidelines

Purpose: The Committee for the Control and Supervision of Experiments on Animals (CCSEA) aims to uphold the humane treatment of animals in experimental research by enforcing strict regulatory oversight and supervision. The committee's primary focus is to minimize unnecessary pain, suffering, and distress, thereby fostering ethical and responsible scientific practices involving the use of animals. By acting as a regulatory body, the CCSEA ensures that the welfare of animals is prioritized and safeguarded in research environments.

Mandate: The mandate of the CCSEA is to ensure strict compliance with ethical guidelines and legal requirements pertaining to animal experimentation. This involves monitoring and evaluating research practices to ensure that they adhere to the established standards of animal welfare. The committee is tasked with reviewing and approving research protocols, conducting inspections, and providing guidance to researchers to ensure that all experiments are conducted responsibly and ethically.

Principles: The CCSEA operates on a set of core principles aimed at promoting respect for animal life. This includes minimizing pain and distress experienced by animals during experiments. Researchers are required to employ the principles of the Refinement, Reduction, and Replacement (the three Rs) to ensure that animal use is justified, the number of animals used is minimized, and procedures are refined to enhance animal welfare.

Scope: The guidelines and oversight of the CCSEA extend to all researchers and facilities engaged in the use of animals for scientific, educational, and medical purposes. This includes universities, research institutions, and private laboratories. The CCSEA functions as the Institutional Animal Ethics Committee (IAEC) at the local level, providing localized oversight and ensuring that all animal use within institutions is in compliance with national and international standards.

Commitment: The CCSEA is committed to fostering a culture of accountability and ethical responsibility in scientific research. This involves continuous education and training for researchers, promoting transparency in research practices, and encouraging the development and adoption of alternatives to animal testing. The committee is dedicated to advancing science in a manner that respects animal welfare and upholds the highest ethical standards.

Sincere attempts have been made to clearly explain the theoretical parts of the pharmaceutical practical components, accompanied by flowcharts and illustrations. Giving pupils comprehensive knowledge of the subject in an easy-to-understand format is the main goal of this book. The challenges that students typically encounter have been taken into consideration. The book's noteworthy aspects are:

1. It covers every subject listed in the Pharmacy Council of India's "Bachelor of Pharmacy (B. Pharm) course regulations 2014."

2. The language used is modest and eloquent.

We earnestly believe and apprehend that the brilliant budding students of pharmacy (Degree Program) in all Indian universities will definitely find this compilation extremely useful to provide them with sufficient deliberation, understanding, and in-depth knowledge on the subject.

We are grateful to Editorial Manager Publications, Bentham Science Publishers, Sharjah, U.A.E., for all their efforts in publishing this book.

Suggestions and comments are always welcome, and they shall be gratefully acknowledged.

Suman Kamlesh Rattan
Department of Pharmacy
A Central University
Guru Ghasidas Vishwavidyalaya
Bilaspur, Chhattisgarh 495009, India

Kedar Prasad Meena
Department of Pharmacy,
A Central University,
Guru Ghasidas Vishwavidyalaya
Bilaspur, Chhattisgarh 495009, India

&

Venu Anand Das Vaishnav
Department of Pharmacy (Neuropharmacology)
A Central University, Guru Ghasidas Vishwavidyalaya
Bilaspur, Chhattisgarh 495009, India

CHAPTER 1

Introduction to Experimental Pharmacology

OBJECTIVE

To study the general introduction of pharmacology and experimental pharmacology.

Pharmacology is a branch of science that is concerned with the investigation of medications. The word "pharmacology" originates from the Greek words "*Pharmakon*" (a drug or poison) and "*logos*" (discourse). It provides information on the genesis, background, physiochemical properties, and physiological properties, as well as the mechanism of action, distribution, metabolism, excretion, and absorption of drugs. Chemicals known as drugs are employed in the diagnosis, treatment, and prevention of disease in both mammals and humans. The word "drug" originates from the French word "*drogue*" meaning "herb." Within basic medical sciences, the field of experimental pharmacology is relatively recent. Advancements in electrophysiology, biochemistry, molecular biology, and the use of digital recording equipment and software have increased and improved the potential for pharmacology in experimental studies.

The major targets of experimental pharmacology are:

1. To identify a treatment drug that is suitable for individual usage
2. To investigate the toxicity of a drug
3. To investigate the mechanism of action of drugs

There are two primary phases of experimental pharmacology, as it entails finding new therapeutic agents or analyzing how already existing ones work [1].

Preclinical experimental pharmacology is the study of novel chemical structures, their identification and optimization, and their biological activities in animal tissues or organs.

Clinical pharmacology is the study of pharmacological safety, effectiveness, and pharmacokinetics in humans through the testing of pharmaceuticals on patients and volunteers.

Pharmacokinetics is the study of drug distribution, metabolism, excretion, and absorption, which shows the effects of medications on the body [2].

Pharmacodynamics is an exploration of the drugs' mechanisms of action and sites of action, or what the drugs do to the body [3].

Absorption is the intake of a drug that enters the bloodstream or systemic circulation at the point of administration, which shows a systemic action.

Distribution is the traveling of a drug from the systemic circulation to different organs, tissues, muscles, fat, and so forth.

Metabolism is the transformation of a drug into its excretory form.

Elimination is the process of removal of a drug from the body.

Bioavailability is the percentage of an administered dose of an unaltered medication that enters the bloodstream.

Drugs' active components are helpful in the diagnosis, treatment, mitigation, and prevention of any illness or condition in both humans and animals.

Medicine is a material that contains lubricants, binders, sweeteners, and other additives along with the active component and is used to deliver drugs in a stable and acceptable form.

Neuropharmacology is the study of the effects of medication on the functioning of the central and peripheral nervous systems [4].

Pharmacogenetics is the clinical testing of genetic variation that gives rise to differing responses to drugs.

Posology is the study of drug dosage; it depends upon various factors like age, climate, weight, sex, and so on [5].

Pharmacovigilance is described as the study and practice of identifying, evaluating, and comprehending negative impacts.

Side effects are unintended but predictable consequences of a medication or medical procedure.

Adverse effects are secondary effects that are defined as typically undesirable and unsuitable responses.

CONCLUSION

The experiment provided a comprehensive introduction to experimental pharmacology, equipping students with theoretical and practical knowledge of drug evaluation using laboratory models. By exploring key concepts like animal model selection, drug administration, and data interpretation, students can gain insights into the methodologies used to study pharmacological effects. The ethical aspects, such as humane treatment of animals and compliance with CCSEA guidelines, were emphasized to ensure responsible research practices. The introduction to instruments like the Rota Rod and organ bath demonstrated their relevance in assessing the actions of drugs. This foundational experiment underscored the importance of experimental pharmacology in bridging the gap between basic research and clinical application. It will prepare students for advanced studies in pharmacology, emphasizing accuracy, reproducibility, and ethical considerations essential for conducting meaningful preclinical research.

REFERENCES

[1]   Shankar P, Banga H, Dixit RK. Practical manual of experimental and clinical pharmacology. Asian man (The) - An International Journal. 2013; 7(1and2): 232.
[http://dx.doi.org/10.5958/j.0975-6884.7.1X.032]

[2]   Csajka C, Verotta D. Pharmacokinetic-pharmacodynamic modelling: history and perspectives. J Pharmacokinet Pharmacodyn 2006; 33(3): 227-79.
[http://dx.doi.org/10.1007/s10928-005-9002-0] [PMID: 16404503]

[3]   Sheiner LB, Steimer JL. Pharmacokinetic/pharmacodynamic modeling in drug development. Annu Rev Pharmacol Toxicol 2000; 40(1): 67-95.
[http://dx.doi.org/10.1146/annurev.pharmtox.40.1.67] [PMID: 10836128]

[4]   Heal DJ, Cheetham SC, Smith SL. The neuropharmacology of ADHD drugs *in vivo*: Insights on efficacy and safety. Neuropharmacology 2009; 57(7-8): 608-18.
[http://dx.doi.org/10.1016/j.neuropharm.2009.08.020] [PMID: 19761781]

[5]   Guo MY, Cheng J, Etminan M, Zafari Z, Maberley D. One year effectiveness study of intravitreal aflibercept in neovascular age-related macular degeneration: a meta-analysis. Acta Ophthalmol 2019; 97(1): e1-7.
[http://dx.doi.org/10.1111/aos.13825] [PMID: 30030923]

CHAPTER 2

Instruments Used in Experimental Pharmacology Laboratory

OBJECTIVE

To study the commonly used instruments in experimental pharmacology.

Despite the rapid advancements in electronic equipment and recording systems, research laboratories and institutions still employ them. In experimental pharmacy, certain standard tools are utilized. Even with the leaps in electronic equipment and recording systems, traditional tools continue to hold their ground in research labs and institutions. In experimental pharmacology, several standard tools are essential for the precise and accurate conduct of experiments.

Actophotometer

An actophotometer is a tool used to quantify the locomotor activity of small animals, most commonly rats, in behavior pharmacology (Fig. **1**) [1]. It is an essential technique for pharmacological research, especially when examining how different drugs affect the central nervous system (CNS). When an animal walks through the chamber, the infrared light beams within the chamber are disrupted. The photoelectric sensors translate the incident into an electronic signal and identify each disruption. The signals are routed through a computerized counter, which logs each disruption as an activity unit. The animal's locomotor activity is measured as the total number of interruptions over a given time period.

Rota rod Apparatus

The rotarod test is a behavioral assessment that utilizes a rotating rod to evaluate motor function in rodents (Fig. **2**) [2]. The test gauges important factors, including balance duration (in seconds) and sustained performance. The primary objectives of the test apparatus are to evaluate balance, grip strength, and motor coordination in subjects, particularly in the context of experimental drug trials and post-traumatic brain injury assessments in pharmacological studies.

Suman Kamlesh Rattan, Kedar Prasad Meena & Venu Anand Das Vaishnav

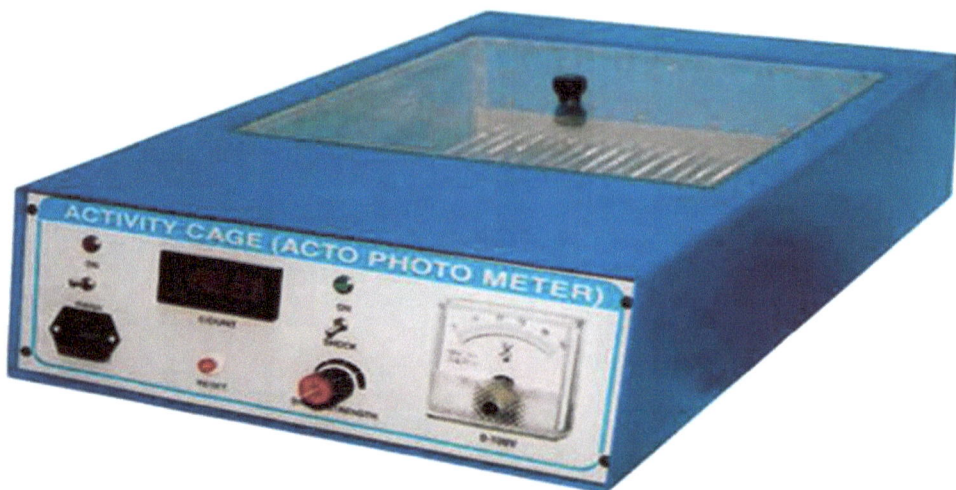

Fig. (1). Actophotometer.

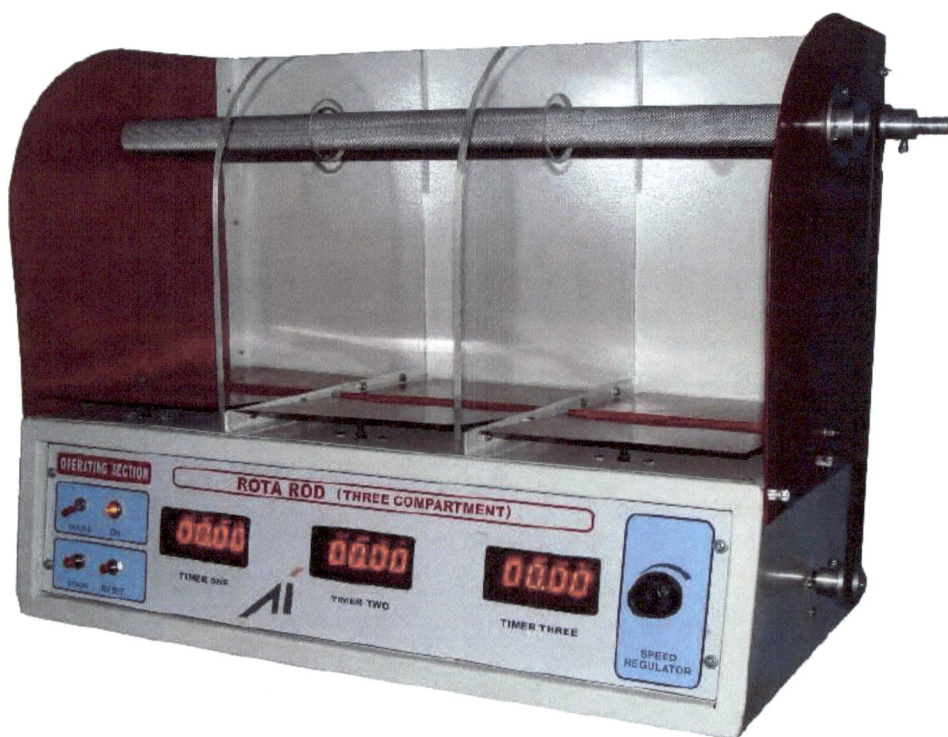

Fig. (2). Rota rod apparatus.

Electro-Convulsometer

Electrical stimulation causes seizures, which are subsequently inhibited by systemic anticonvulsant medication (Fig. **3**) [3]. It is possible to study various forms of epilepsy in animal models in labs. Maximum electroshock causes a convulsion in the lab animals. The categories of MES convulsions are tonic flexion, tonic extensor, tonic fission, clonic convulsion, stupor, and recovery/death.

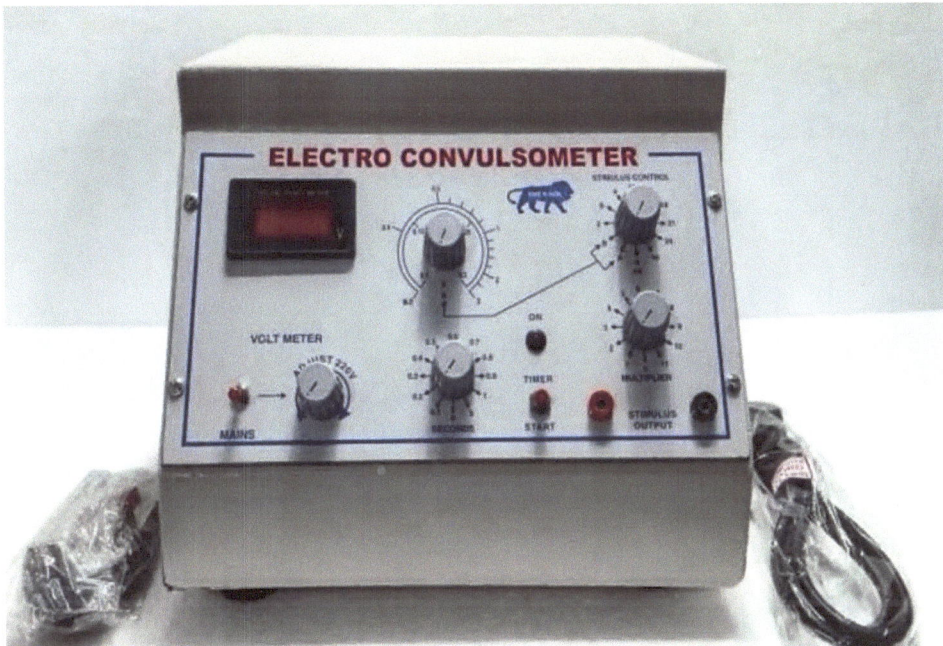

Fig. (3). Electro-Convulsometer.

Eddy's Hotplate

As a source of pain or a stimulant, we use the hotplate. A hotplate is an apparatus with an outside surface and a plate that is heated by an inside heating coil (Fig. **4**) [4]. Mice are the most suitable animal species for this experiment. Mouse species are singled out on this device, which maintains temperature; an analgesic extends the duration in a steady manner using a regulator. Preheating surface with a solid-state and microcontroller-based temperature controller for digital temperature indication allows for precise setting of surface temperature. Animal responses like jumping or licking their paws are recorded at a constant temperature of 550 degrees Celsius. Eddy's hot plate test is used for the evaluation of the analgesic effect of drugs.

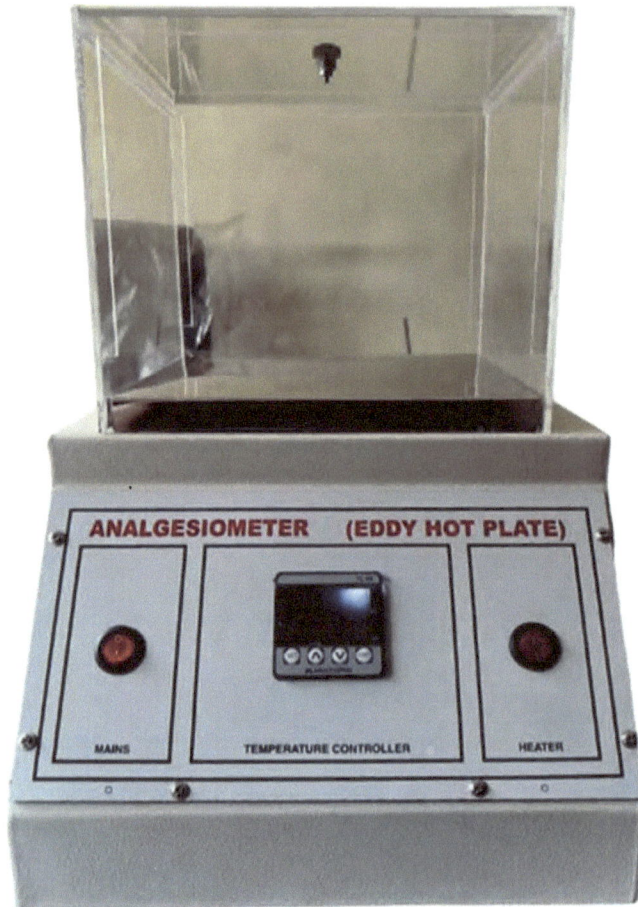

Fig. (4). Eddy's hot plate.

Analgesiometer

An analgesiometer is used to gauge an animal's pain threshold or tolerance. It is frequently employed in studies to assess the efficiency of analgesic (pain-relieving) medications (Fig. **5**) [5]. Analgesiometers come in several forms that are intended to provide an animal with a regulated, measurable stimulus (such as heat, pressure, or electric shock) and then measure the animal's reaction, which represents the amount of pain the animal is feeling. There are different types of analgesiometers, such as hot plate analgesiometer, tail-flick analgesiometer, radiant heat analgesiometer, mechanical or pressure analgesiometer (Randall-Selitto test), and electric shock analgesiometer.

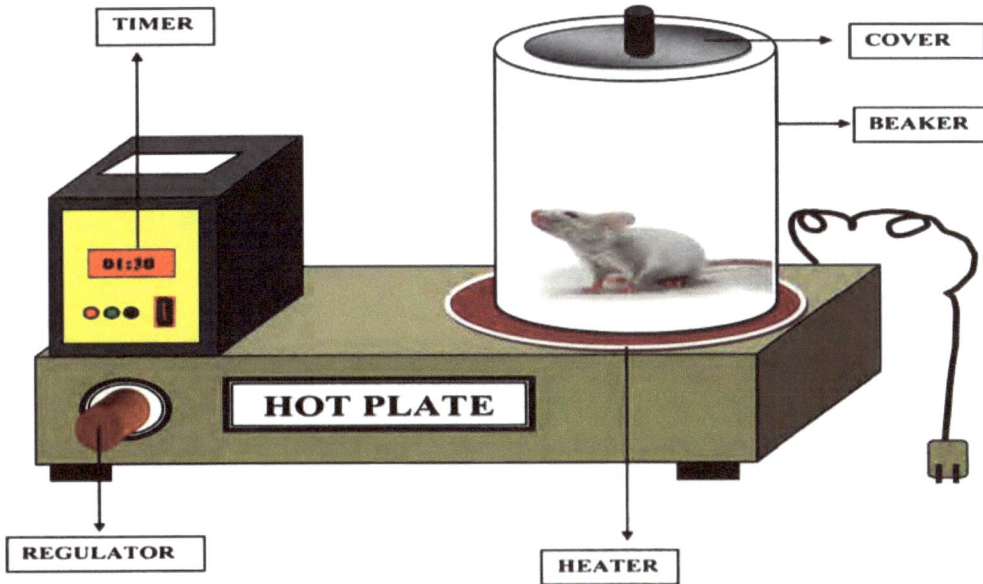

Fig. (5). Analgesiometer.

Elevated Plus Maze

A popular experimental apparatus in behavioral neuroscience, the Elevated Plus Maze (EPM), is a tool used to investigate rodent anxiety, mostly in rats and mice (Fig. **6**) [6]. The EPM is an effective method for determining whether pharmaceutical drugs have anxiolytic or anxiogenic effects because it utilizesmice's innate aversion to open spaces and elevated areas. An equipment in the form of a plus sign, with two open arms and two closed arms, each with an open ceiling, raised 40–70 cm off the ground, makes up the test setup. An increase in the percentage of time spent in the open arms (time in open arms/total time in open or closed arms) and an increase in the percentage of entries into the open arms are indicators of decreased anxiety in the plus maze (total entries into closed or open arms; entries into open arms). The total number of limb entries and the quantity of closed-arm entries are typically used as indicators of overall action.

The EPM is widely used in pharmacological research to evaluate the anxiolytic or anxiogenic effects of drugs. It is also used to study the impact of genetic modifications and neurological conditions on anxiety-related behavior.

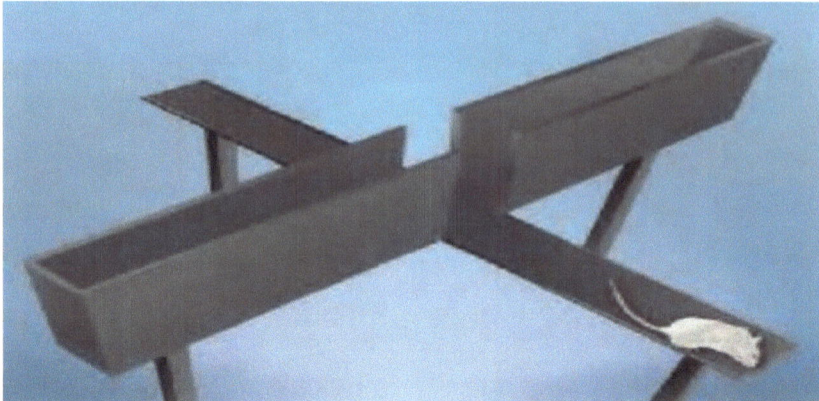

Fig. (6). Elevated plus maze.

Organ bath

Student organ bath: This type of tissue bath is used to hold animal tissue, which is used to examine the effects of drugs (Fig. **7**) [7]. Rudolph Magnus created this initially in 1904. The glass tissue bath or inner organ has a volume ranging from 10 to 50 milliliters.

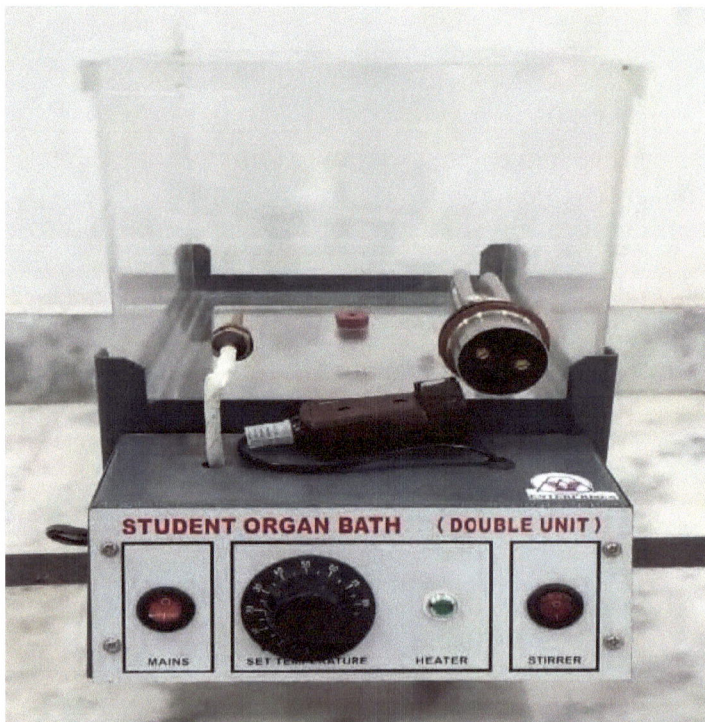

Fig. (7). Organ bath.

In essence, the organ bath consists of:

• An outer jacket composed of Perspex, glass, or steel.
• A heating rod with thermostat control.
• A stirrer to keep the water in the outer jacket at a constant temperature.
• Glass delivery or oxygen tube that doubles as a tissue holder.
• A glass coil with a physiological salt solution linked to one end.

A student organ bath with two inner tissue bath units are referred to as a double unit organ bath.

CONCLUSION

The experiment demonstrated the functionality and uses of instruments routinely used in experimental pharmacology. The Rota Rod apparatus, actophotometer, plethysmograph, and organ bath helped students develop key technical skills and an awareness of the role that these instruments play in evaluating the effects of drugs. This was accomplished by offering students hands-on training with this equipment. Through the use of this experiment, a basic knowledge base was established for further pharmacological studies. The experiment also highlighted the importance of integrating technology and methodology in order to enhance research in the field of drug development and testing.

REFERENCES

[1]   Patel R, Agrawal S, Jain NS. Stimulation of dorsal hippocampal histaminergic transmission mitigates the expression of ethanol withdrawal-induced despair in mice. Alcohol 2021; 96: 1-14.
[http://dx.doi.org/10.1016/j.alcohol.2021.06.002] [PMID: 34228989]

[2]   Rozas G, Guerra MJ, Labandeira-García JL. An automated rotarod method for quantitative drug-free evaluation of overall motor deficits in rat models of parkinsonism. Brain Res Brain Res Protoc 1997; 2(1): 75-84.
[http://dx.doi.org/10.1016/S1385-299X(97)00034-2] [PMID: 9438075]

[3]   Junnarkar AY, Singh PP. Antagonism of clonidine-induced hypothermia by alpha adrenoceptor antagonists in electrically stimulated mice. Pharmacol Res Commun 1988; 20(6): 451-63.
[http://dx.doi.org/10.1016/S0031-6989(88)80074-2] [PMID: 2901758]

[4]   Cintolesi C, Petronio A, Armenio V. Large-eddy simulation of thin film evaporation and condensation from a hot plate in enclosure: First order statistics. Int J Heat Mass Transf 2016; 101: 1123-37.
[http://dx.doi.org/10.1016/j.ijheatmasstransfer.2016.06.006]

[5]   Malairajan P, Geetha Gopalakrishnan , Narasimhan S, Jessi Kala Veni K. Analgesic activity of some Indian medicinal plants. J Ethnopharmacol 2006; 106(3): 425-8.
[http://dx.doi.org/10.1016/j.jep.2006.03.015] [PMID: 16647234]

[6]   Rodgers RJ, Dalvi A. Anxiety, defence and the elevated plus-maze. Neurosci Biobehav Rev 1997; 21(6): 801-10.
[http://dx.doi.org/10.1016/S0149-7634(96)00058-9] [PMID: 9415905]

[7]   Rendig SV, Amsterdam E. A multitissue organ bath evaluated using new rabbit papillary muscle isolation methods. Pharmacology 1992; 44(3): 169-76.
[http://dx.doi.org/10.1159/000138910] [PMID: 1579599]

CHAPTER 3

Study of Common Laboratory Animals

OBJECTIVE

To study about common laboratory animals.

Mouse (*Mus musculus*)

Surplus albino mice (*Mus musculus*) are frequently employed (Fig. **8**) [1] as they are comparable, affordable, tiny, and manageable.

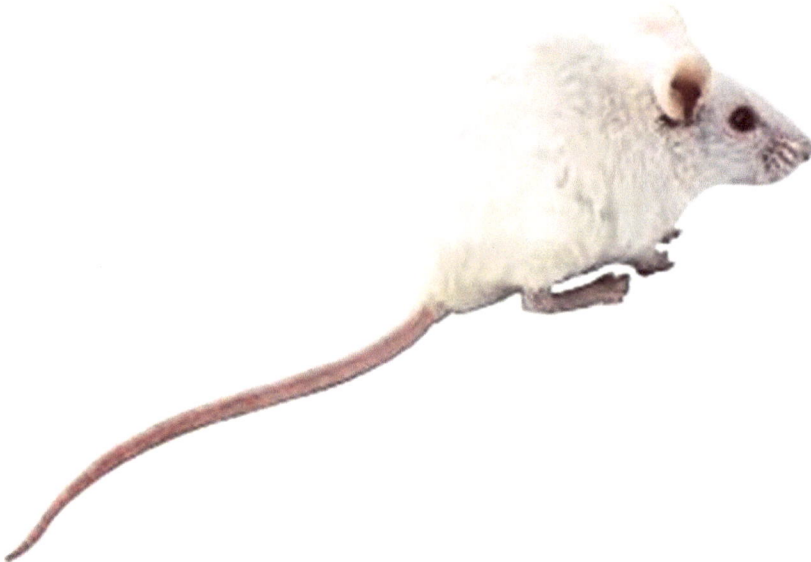

Fig. (8). Mouse (*Mus musculus*).

Common behavior:

- Timid
- Social
- Territorial
- Nocturnal
- Rarely aggressive when handled properly

Adult weight range for experimental use is 20 to 25 gm; two months is the minimum age for experimentation.

- Acute and sub-acute toxicity are the focus of toxicology studies.
- Insulin bioassay
- Analgesic screening
- Research pertaining to cancer and genetics

Rat (*Rattus norvegicus*)

Wistar strain rats are frequently employed (Fig. **9**) [2]. Commonly employed strains include Sprague-Dawley rats.

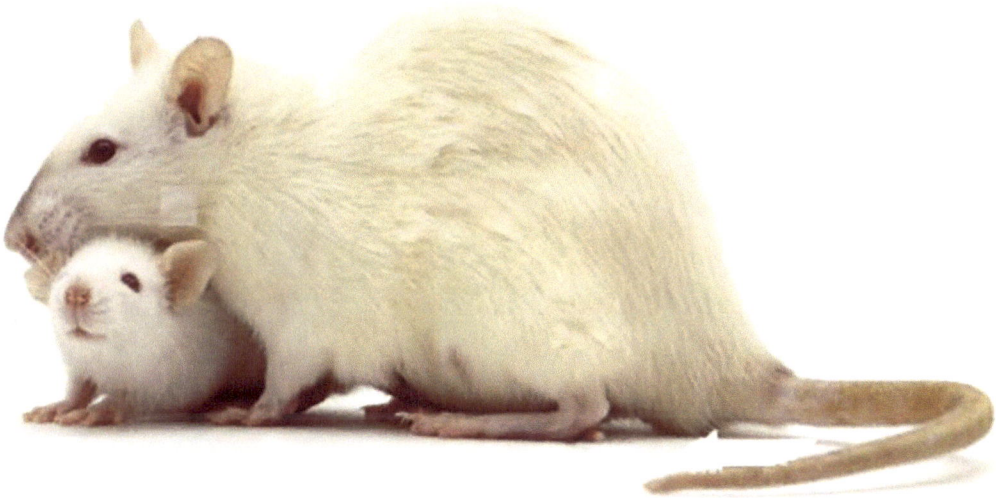

Fig. (9). Rat (*Rattus norvegicus*).

- Because of the diminutive size in relation to other animals, a tiny amount of medication is given.
- The drug can be administered orally because of the lack of a vomiting center.
- The tonsils and gall bladder are absent.
- Pancreatectomy is difficult to achieve because of the widespread nature of the pancreas.
- A distinct line exists between the stomach's fundus and pylorus sections.

For experimental use, adult weight range is 200-250 mg; one and a half months of age is appropriate for trials.

- Psychopharmacology
- Study of analgesic and anticonvulsant drugs
- Oestrus cycle study
- Gastric acid secretion study
- Chronic study on blood pressure

Guinea pig (*Cavia porcellus*)

The guinea pig is calm and particularly vulnerable to tuberculosis and anaphylaxis. Theyreact strongly to histamine and penicillin (Fig. **10**) [3].

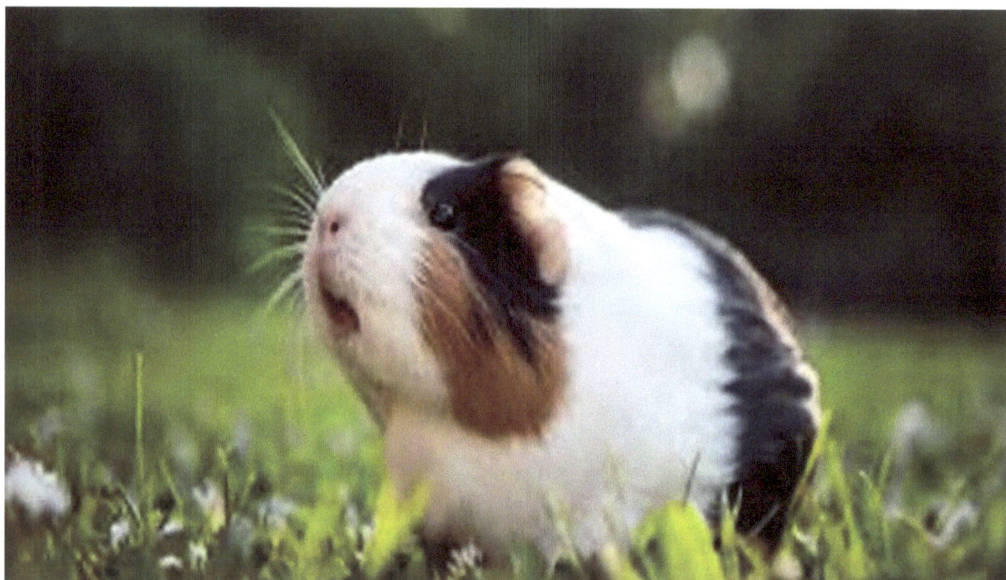

Fig. (10). Guinea pig (*Cavia porcellus*).

Experimental use: The adult weight range for the experiment is 400-600g; the age range is two months

- Evaluation of bronchodilators
- Studies on immunology
- Studies on the oestrus cycle
- Studies on mast cells

Rabbit (*Oryctolagus cuniculus*)

Oryctolagus cuniculus, commonly known as the European rabbit, is a species that has significant ecological, cultural, agricultural, and research relevance (Fig. **11**) [4]. (Adult weight ranges from 1.3-2 kg)

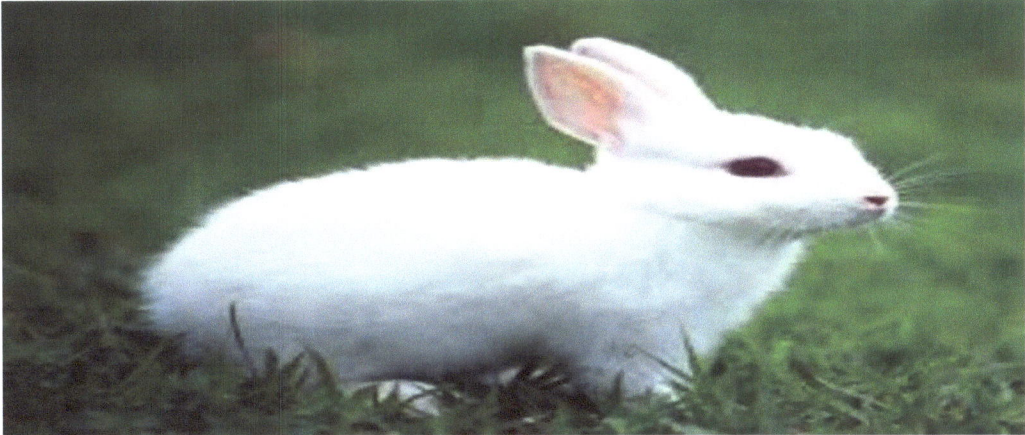

Fig. (11). Rabbit (*Oryctolagus cuniculus*).

Experimental use:

- Pyrogenic testing
- Test for irritation
- Study on pharmacokinetics
- Antidiabetic bioassay
- Genomic screening of embryos

Hamster (*Circetulus grisceus*)

Hamsters have a small body with legs and a tail. The fur is short, silky, and dense, covering loose skin. The cheek pouches are noticeable and extend to the shoulder area (Fig. **12**) [5].

Experimental use: Adult weight range is 80-90g; an age of 1 month is appropriate for the experiment

- Due to its 1000 chromosome count, Chinese hamsters are beneficial for cytological investigations.
- Prostaglandin bioassay
- Studies on diabetes mellitus

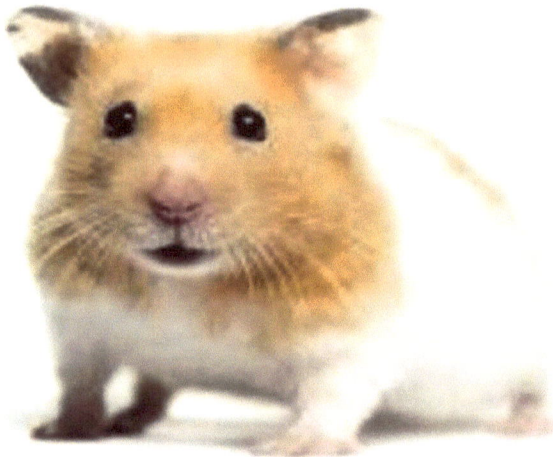

Fig. (12). Hamster (*Circetulus grisceus*).

Frog (*Rana tigrina*)

A common animal used in physiology, toxicology, and pharmacology, this species has been used in experiments for over 200 years; it is an amphibian that is safe to handle, cannot be bred in a lab, and contains the neurotransmitter adrenaline in the sympathetic nervous system (Fig. **13**) [6].

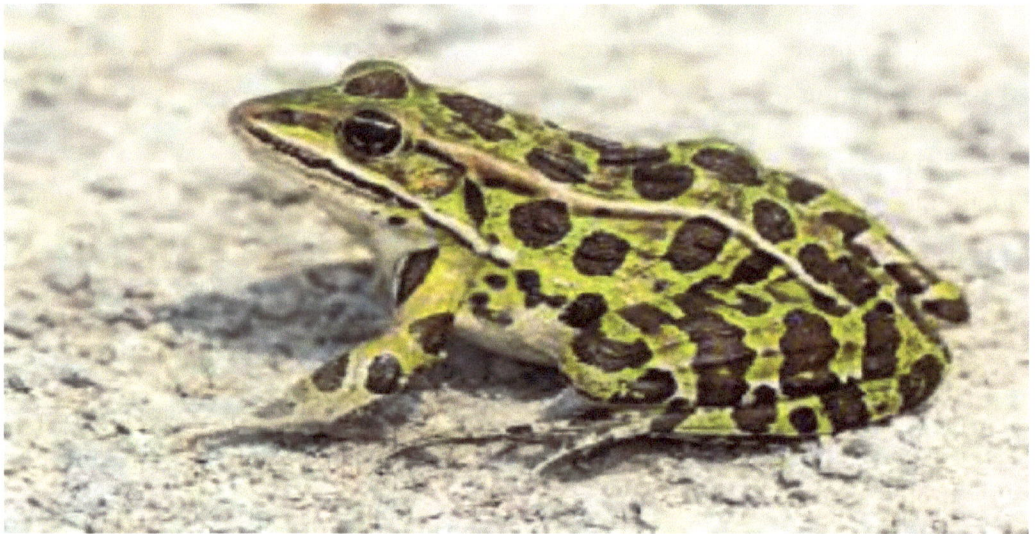

Fig. (13). Frog (*Rana tigrina*).

Experimental use:

• Study on isolated tissues, such as the heart and the rectus abdominis muscle
• Study on drugs that affect the central nervous system
• Pharmaceutical research on the neuromuscular junction

Other Animals

Drug pharmacological studies are also conducted on dogs (Fig. **14**) [7], cats (Fig. **15**) [8], and monkeys (Fig. **16**) [9]. In the past, blood pressure investigations were frequently conducted on cats and dogs. Their use is now limited, nevertheless. However, the only strain that the FDA has authorized for preclinical research is beagle dogs for testing novel pharmaceuticals.

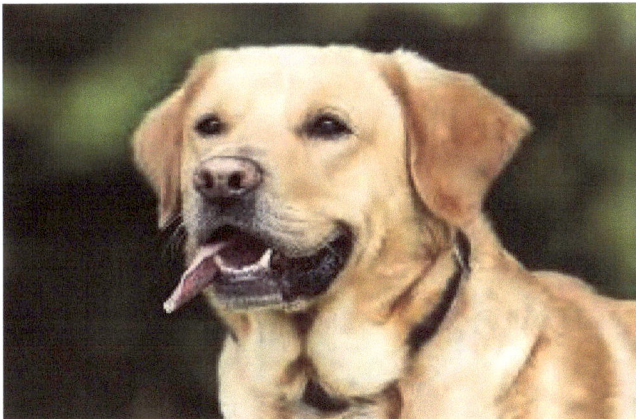

Fig. (14). Dog (*Canis lupus familiaris*).

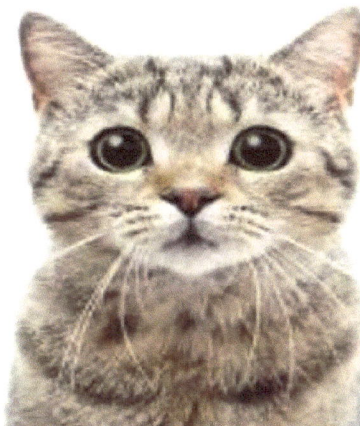

Fig. (15). Cat (*Felis catus*).

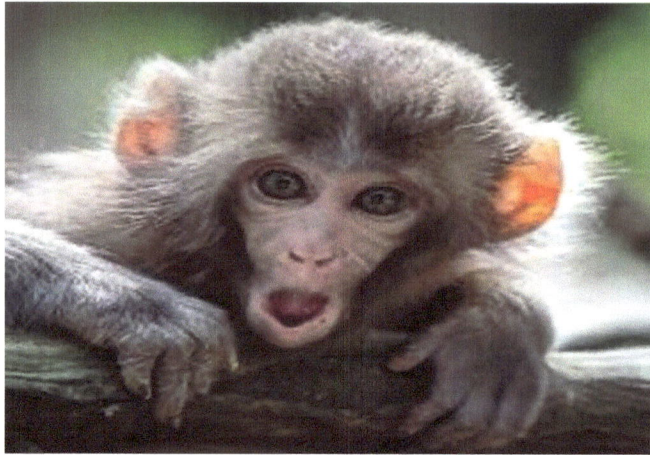

Fig. (16). Monkey (*Macaca mulatta*).

CONCLUSION

With the help of this study, students were successfully introduced to the common laboratory animals used in research. The study focused on the biological characteristics, behavior, and care requirements of these animals. The selection of acceptable models for experiments and the guaranteeing of accurate results both require an understanding of the characteristics and requirements that are peculiar to a species. The relevance of humane practices in animal research was brought to light by the reinforcement of proper handling skills and the adherence to ethical guidelines. The experiment highlighted the importance of ensuring the well-being of laboratory animals, as this has a direct bearing on the reliability and repeatability of scientific findings. It is essential for researchers to have this basic knowledge in order to design and carry out studies in a responsible manner, ensuring compliance with regulatory standards and cultivating a culture of ethical research. The research also highlighted the significant contribution that laboratory animals make to the advancement of human and veterinary medicine, as well as the vital role that they play in the progression of scientific research.

REFERENCES

[1]   Camus MC, Chapman MJ, Forgez P, Laplaud PM. Distribution and characterization of the serum lipoproteins and apoproteins in the mouse, Mus musculus. J Lipid Res 1983; 24(9): 1210-28.
[http://dx.doi.org/10.1016/S0022-2275(20)37904-9] [PMID: 6631247]

[2]   Eilam D, Golani I. Home base behavior of rats (*Rattus norvegicus*) exploring a novel environment. Behav Brain Res 1989; 34(3): 199-211.
[http://dx.doi.org/10.1016/S0166-4328(89)80102-0] [PMID: 2789700]

[3]   Evans E, Benato L. Pain management in pet guinea pigs (*Cavia porcellus*): a review of limitations of current knowledge and practice. Vet Anaesth Analg 2024.
[PMID: 39924411]

[4]   Naff KA, Craig S. The Domestic Rabbit, *Oryctolagus Cuniculus*. The Laboratory Rabbit, Guinea Pig,

Hamster, and Other Rodents. Elsevier 2012; pp. 157-63.
[http://dx.doi.org/10.1016/B978-0-12-380920-9.00006-7]

[5]   Feeney WP. The Chinese or Striped-Back Hamster. The Laboratory Rabbit, Guinea Pig, Hamster, and Other Rodents. Elsevier 2012; pp. 907-22.
        [http://dx.doi.org/10.1016/B978-0-12-380920-9.00035-3]

[6]   Gambhir SS, Tripathi RM, Das PK. Studies on mast cells of Rana tigrina. Eur J Pharmacol 1978; 49(4): 437-40.
        [http://dx.doi.org/10.1016/0014-2999(78)90318-7] [PMID: 668813]

[7]   Galibert F, Quignon P, Hitte C, André C. Toward understanding dog evolutionary and domestication history. C R Biol 2011; 334(3): 190-6.
        [http://dx.doi.org/10.1016/j.crvi.2010.12.011] [PMID: 21377613]

[8]   Turner DC. A review of over three decades of research on cat-human and human-cat interactions and relationships. Behav Processes 2017; 141(Pt 3): 297-304.
        [http://dx.doi.org/10.1016/j.beproc.2017.01.008] [PMID: 28119016]

[9]   Jana S, Maqbool M, Yan X, *et al.* Development and evaluation in rat and monkey of a candidate homochiral radioligand for PET studies of brain receptor interacting protein kinase 1: [^{18} F](*S*)-1-- 5-(3-Fluorophenyl)-4,5-dihydro-1 *H* -pyrazol-1-yl)-2,2-dimethylpropan-1-one. ACS Chem Neurosci 2025; 16(2): 203-22.
        [http://dx.doi.org/10.1021/acschemneuro.4c00715] [PMID: 39745023]

CHAPTER 4

Maintenance of Laboratory Animals as per CCSEA Guidelines

OBJECTIVE

To study the maintenance of laboratory animals as per CCSEA guidelines.

The objective of Good Laboratory Practices (GLP) for animal facilities is to ensure the welfare and high standard of care for the animals utilized in research studies.

Goal

These guidelines aim to support the humane treatment of animals utilized in behavioral and biological investigations and testing, primarily by offering guidelines that will improve animal welfare and quality in the effort to expand biological information relevant to both humans and animals [1].

Veterinary Care

- It is the duty of a veterinarian or someone with knowledge or expertise in laboratory animal sciences and medicine to offer adequate veterinary care.
- Someone other than a veterinarian must observe animals on a daily basis; but, a system of open and continuous communication ought to be implemented to ensure that timely and reliable information on issues with animal health, behavior, and well-being is sent to the attending veterinary physician.
- Additionally, veterinarians can also assist the organization in creating suitable policies and procedures for secondary veterinary services, like the application of suitable disease prevention and control techniques (*e.g.*, vaccination and prophylaxis, disease surveillance and observation, seclusion, and monitoring), surgical and post-operative treatment, diagnosis, and management of both injuries and illnesses. They can also do this by analyzing proposals and procedures, animal husbandry, and the well-being of animals, as well as keeping an eye on the containment of occupational health risks, developing initiatives to control zoonosis, and overseeing animal care and cleanliness. Established conditions dictate whether full-time, part-time, or consultative veterinarian care is required [2].

Acquisition of Animals

All animals (including sheep, goats, cattle, buffalo, pigs, and horses, among others) must be legally obtained in accordance with the CCSEA regulations. Dogs and small animals can be obtained from licensed breeders. Large animals can be obtained from farmers, or under the direction of the department of wildlife, similar to how macaques are treated. Cats are useful for breeding purposes. It is possible to transport rats from overseas following the acquisition of the required Director General of Foreign Trade (DGFT) license for import. Animal quality should be evaluated before purchasing by conducting a health surveillance program for purchased animals. It is also important to consider the modes of transportation. Animals should be quarantined and stabilized in accordance with protocols suitable for the species and situation, and every shipment of animals should be examined to ensure that procurement requirements are met [3].

Quarantine, Stabilization, and Separation

- When an animal is placed in quarantine, it is kept apart from other animals in the facility until its health and maybe its microbiological status are established. An efficient quarantine reduces the possibility of germs entering an established colony. Small laboratory animals are quarantined for one week to one month, while larger animals (cats, dogs, monkeys, *etc.*) are quarantined for up to six weeks. However, the duration depends on the kind of infection or probable infection found in animals.
- To assist in reducing human exposure to zoonotic illnesses, non-human primates should be placed under effective quarantine. Depending on how the TB test turns out, the duration can range from two to three months. Worldwide, macaques that test positive for tuberculosis at least twice or those who exhibit symptoms of illness or weight loss are euthanized to avoid transfer of tuberculosis to employees and other macaques.
- Newly arrived animals should be allowed a period for physiological, psychological, and nutritional stability before being used, regardless of the length of the quarantine. The period and type of animal transportation used, the species involved, and the stabilization period will all affect how long it takes, as well as the animals' intended purpose.
- To prevent the spread of diseases between species, reduce anxiety, and avoid any physiological and behavioral changes brought on by interspecies conflict, it is advised that animals be physically separated by species.
- Different species are typically housed in distinct rooms, cages with filtered air or separate ventilation, and isolators. It is permissible in certain cases to keep different species in the same room, such as when they are behaviorally compatible and share a comparable pathogenic status. Other workers should be

prohibited from entering the facility unless absolutely necessary, and once they have handled these sick animals, they should not handle any other animals there. A separate set of professionals should be designated to care for these diseased animals.

Monitoring, Diagnosis, Therapy, and Disease Control

- Animal house workers should keep an eye out for any signs of disease, injury, or unusual behavior in all of the animals. This should ideally happen every day, although there are times when more frequent observations are necessary, such as after surgery or in cases where the animal is unwell or physically deficient. Appropriate techniques for illness surveillance and diagnosis must be implemented.
- In order to guarantee the proper and timely provision of veterinary medical treatment, post-mortem examination should be done whenever an animal exhibits signs of disease, suffering, or other abnormalities in their general health as soon as possible. Animals that exhibit symptoms of a communicable illness ought to be kept apart from the colony's healthy animals. When non-human primates are exposed to an infectious pathogen, such as *Mycobacterium tuberculosis*, the group should be segregated and maintained together for diagnosis and treatment to control the spread of the disease. Animals with infectious illnesses, such as tuberculosis, *etc.*, must be put to death immediately to stop them from spreading to other animals and even to animal handlers.
- For newly arrived animals, isolation, quarantine, and stabilization programs are required to give time for a health status evaluation, help them recuperate from the stress of transportation, and provide them time to become acclimated to their new environment. The scope of these initiatives is determined by several elements, such as the animals' species, origin, and intended purpose. For certain animals, such as rodents that come from trustworthy sources and whose health status is known, a quick examination upon arrival might be sufficient. For animals, such as agricultural animals, nonhuman primates, wild creatures, canines, rodents, and rabbits, that are free of particular pathogens, it is necessary to follow isolation and quarantine protocols.
- Vaccinations, treatments for ecto- and endoparasites, and other disease management methods are examples of preventive medicine programs that should be started in accordance with current veterinary medical standards suitable for the specific species and source.
- Animals that are transgenic or mutant may be more vulnerable to illness and may need more care to maintain their health. Standard operating procedures, containment/isolation devices, and facility design elements are a few examples of systems used to stop the transmission of illness. To stop the spread of animal diseases, personnel involved in research and animal care must receive proper

training.

- A veterinarian's primary duty is disease surveillance, which should involve routinely checking animals in the colony for the existence of microbiological and parasitic pathogens that could cause overt or covert disease. Furthermore, transplantable cancers, as well as tissues, cells, and fluids, should be checked for parasitic or pathogenic organisms that could result in illness in domestic animals. Vet opinion is also crucial, as well as the kind, origin, purpose, and quantity of animals kept and employed in the amenities.

- Services for diagnostic laboratories must be offered and utilized as needed. Necropsy, histology, microbiology, clinical pathology, serology, parasitology, and other standard or specialist laboratory tests should all be included in the laboratory services, as needed. It is not essential that the animal facility have access to all of these services (Facilities from other laboratories with the necessary equipment are permitted).

- Animals that have infectious or contagious diseases need to be kept apart from other animals by keeping them in isolation rooms or other spaces that are suitable for containing the agents of concern. Under specific conditions, when a whole population of animals is believed or confirmed to be exposed to infection, it might be acceptable to keep them together for the duration necessary to complete a project, to carry out further control procedures, or for diagnosis and treatment

- After diagnosing an animal illness or damage, the veterinarian must be authorized to undertake the proper therapy or restraint methods, such as euthanasia, following consultation with a minimum of one additional veterinarian, if required. The main investigator and the veterinarian should talk over the situation in order to determine a course of action that will best meet the goals of the study. However, if the lead researcher is unavailable or if a consensus cannot be reached, the veterinarian needs to be able to take action to safeguard the health and welfare of the personnel and the institutional animal colony.

Animal Care and Technical Personnel

Support for technical and husbandry aspects is necessary for animal care initiatives. Institutions should provide both formal and on-the-job training, or hire people with experience in laboratory animal research, to ensure the program is implemented successfully (Annexure-7).

Personal Hygiene

- The personnel who work with animals must always keep a high level of personal hygiene. Facilities should be equipped with the proper Personal Protective Equipment (PPE), such as showers, clothes changes, shoes, and so forth.

- Clothing that is appropriate for usage at an animal facility ought to be provided and cleaned by the establishment. On the other hand, clothing that has come into contact with hazardous materials, microbiological agents, or potentially dangerous items should be cleaned in institutional facilities. In many cases, a professional laundry service is suitable. It is appropriate to wear masks, headgear, disposable gloves, jackets, shoe covers, and other protective gear. Staff should change into new clothes as frequently as possible, which is essential for upholding one's personal hygiene. Clothing worn inside the animal quarters is not permitted to be worn outside the animal housing facility.
- Facilities for showering and washing that are suitable for the program should be offered. In animal rooms, staff members should not be allowed to eat, drink, smoke, or wear makeup or fragrances. They should leave the animal quarters or rooms as soon as the task with the animals is finished, and go somewhere else instead, such as outside. They should have access to a separate area or room designated for these uses.

Employing Hazardous Agents in Animal Experiments

- Institutions ought to have guidelines for using dangerous substances in experiments. The majority of institutions of higher learning, research facilities, and the pharmaceutical industry have institutional biosafety committees with members who are educated about dangerous substances and attend to matters of safety. In addition to its existing activities, this committee also examines the concept of testing hazardous compounds on animals.
- Both the Institutional Biosafety Committee and the Institutional Animal Ethics Committee (IAEC) must assess the protocols and the facilities to be used because using animals in such investigations necessitates particular considerations. The disposal of fluids and tissues resulting from such use of animals must also be properly managed in accordance with the institution's established procedures and biosafety standards and controls.

Several Operative Techniques on a Single Animal

- Performing several surgical procedures on a single animal for any kind of study or experiment is prohibited unless specifically approved by the IAEC.
- Individual animals should not be used in more than one experiment, for the same or a different study, without the express permission of the IAEC. Reusing animals appropriately, however, can reduce the total number of animals used in a project, enhance experiment design, and prevent pain or discomfort in other animals. Animals utilized in multiple experiments are allowed to fully recover before the experiment that follows is carried out. Nonetheless, the accompanying veterinarian's certification is necessary before the animal is in the second experiment.

Duration of Experiments

A sufficient rationale must be given before using an animal for research purposes for more than three years.

Physical Restraint

• For the purpose of examination, sample collection, and various other clinical and experimental manipulations, animals can be briefly physically restrained. This can be accomplished manually or by using tools that are suitable in size and form for the animal being handled and that are applied appropriately to lessen stress and shield the animal from injury.
• Extensive animal restraint, such as chairing non-human primates, should be avoided unless it is absolutely required to accomplish the objectives of the investigation. When they are compatible with study aims, less restrictive systems, such as the pole and collar system or the tether system, should be used.

Functional Areas

The need for and feasibility of spaces for distinct service functions depend on a facility's size and design. Adequate space is required to adopt, hold, and separate animals.

These facilities can be:

• Specialist labs
• Individual spaces used for tasks like surgery, critical care, necropsy, radiography, special nutrition preparation, experimental manipulation, treatment, and diagnostic laboratory procedures, also known as containment facilities. These spaces are adjacent to areas where animals live.
• Area for the facility's direction, management, and oversight, as well as restrooms, sinks, lockers, and showers for staff.
• A location where supplies and equipment can be cleaned and sterilized.

Physical Facilities

The efficiency and economy of this activity are largely determined by the physical state and design of the animal facility. The size and layout of an animal facility are determined by the type of research being conducted at the institution, the animals that will be housed there, and the facility's geographic proximity to other institutions. A well-designed and well-maintained facility is a crucial component of proper animal care.

The design and operation of housing facilities should assist in the control of environmental elements to keep out vermin and minimize contamination from animal housing, the supply of food, water, and bedding, as well as from the entrance of animals and other animals.

- Housing facilities need to be kept up and maintained properly. Floors and walls should be made of sturdy materials with surfaces that can be easily cleaned and disinfected.
- Housing facilities ought to be neat and orderly and must be run as hygienically as possible.
- Deodorants should not be used to cover up animal odors because they expose the animals to volatile substances that can change their metabolic processes. Furthermore, deodorants should never be used as a substitute for proper ventilation, cleaning procedures for cages and equipment, and excellent hygiene.

CONCLUSION

The experiment highlighted how important it is to keep laboratory animals in accordance with the rules set forth by the CCSEA in order to protect their welfare and reduce the amount of distress they experience while being used for research. The well-being of laboratory animals is greatly influenced by a number of factors, including the presence of optimal environmental conditions, appropriate housing, and consistent health monitoring, as demonstrated by observations. Compliance with ethical standards not only ensures that humane methods are maintained, but it also improves the reliability of experimental results by lowering the amount of unpredictability that is brought on by stress. The findings of the study highlighted the significance of providing researchers and technicians who are involved in preclinical investigations with the appropriate training in animal care. Adhering to the principles established by the CCSEA develops a culture of responsibility among researchers and guarantees that the use of animals in research is conducted in an ethical manner. The knowledge obtained from this experiment will serve as a foundation for maintaining high standards in animal research, ensuring that both scientific and ethical integrity are maintained.

REFERENCES

[1]   Pandey G, Sharma M. Guidelines of CPCSEA for conducting the experiment on animals. InNational Seminar on Progress in Life Sciences for Human Welfare 2011 researchgate. 2011; 5–6.

[2]   Qadri SSYH, Newcomer CE. Laws, Regulations, and Guidelines Shaping Research Animal Care and Use in India. Laboratory Animals. Elsevier 2014; pp. 219-42.
[http://dx.doi.org/10.1016/B978-0-12-397856-1.00008-8]

[3]   Pereira S, Veeraraghavan P, Ghosh S, Gandhi M. Animal experimentation and ethics in India: the CPCSEA makes a difference. Altern Lab Anim 2004; 32(1_suppl) (1B): 411-5.
[http://dx.doi.org/10.1177/026119290403201s67] [PMID: 23581110]

CHAPTER 5

Commonly Used Laboratory Techniques

OBJECTIVE

To study common laboratory techniques used in animal experiments.

ANESTHESIA IN EXPERIMENTAL ANIMALS

Anesthesia: The loss of feeling, usually brought on by damage to a nerve or receptor, but it can also result from medication use or other medical procedures. **Analgesia:** Pain relief

Tranquilization: A behavioral shift in which the animal exhibits relaxed, environment-indifferent, and frequently pain-indifferent behavior.

Sedation: It causes the animal to be alert and peaceful while having a mild case of CNS depression. Loss of sensation in a specific location is known as local anesthesia.

Insensibility: Anesthesia in a broader but still constrained region.

Basal Anesthesia: A mild form of general anesthesia caused by a pre-anesthetic drug that gets the animal ready for the administration of more drugs or a deeper anesthesia.

General Anesthesia: Total unconsciousness with general anesthesia.

Surface Anesthesia: A state of consciousness combined with a degree of muscle relaxation that permits painless operation. For instance, proparacaine and tetracaine.

Injectable Local Anaesthetics: For gentle and peaceful animals (cattle, sheep), injectable local anesthetics such as proparacaine, lidocaine, mepivacaine, and etiodocaine are used. For the majority of laboratory animals, general anesthesia is the preferred approach. Animals should only be used in experiments for biomedical research if they are cognizant. It is not feasible to conduct the study while the animal is sedated. Conditions for anesthesia should always be selected with the intention of minimizing pain, discomfort, and tension as potential harmful factors on the repeatability of the data and the pharmaceutical outcomes.

GENERAL ANESTHESIA

Preparation: The animal should be made to fast for 12 hrs (Water-fasting ad libitum).

Premedication: To facilitate the administration of the anesthetic and minimize its negative effects. For example, atropine is administered intramuscularly (IM) before general anesthesia to prevent cardiac complications and to reduce salivation (Table **1**) [1].

Table 1. Various medications.

Species	Premedication	Sedation	Short Anaesthesia	Medium Anesthesia	Long Anaesthesia
Rat	Atropine (0.2 s.c.)	Diazepam (2.5 i.m.)	Alfentanyle + Etomidate (0.03+2 i.m.) or inhalation (Isoflurane)	Xylazine + Ketamine (5+100 i.m.) or Phenobarbitone (50 i.p.)	Xylazine + Ketamine (16+100 i.m.)
Mouse	Atropine (0.1-0.25 s.c.)	Diazepam (5 i.p.)	Alfentanyle + Etomidate (0.03+2 i.m.) or inhalation (Isoflurane)	Xylazine + Ketamine (5+100 i.m.) or Phenobarbitone (50 i.p.)	Xylazine + Ketamine (16+100 i.m.)
Hamster	Atropine (0.1-0.2 s.c.)	Diazepam (5 i.p.)	Inhalation (Isoflurane or Ether)	Xylazine + Ketamine (5+50 i.m.) or Phenobarbitone (35 i.p.)	Xylazine + Ketamine (10+200 i.m.)
Guinea Pig	Atropine (0.1-0.2 s.c.)	Diazepam (2.5-5 i.p.)	Inhalation (Isoflurane)	Xylazine + Ketamine (2+80 i.m.)	Xylazine + Ketamine (4+100 i.m.)
Rabbit	Atropine (0.1-0.2 s.c.)	Diazepam (1-5 i.p.)	Inhalation (Isoflurane)	Xylazine + Ketamine (5+25-80 i.m.)	Xylazine + Ketamine (5+100 i.m.)

Xylazine - Administered IM to make the animal calm, dilates the blood vessels.

COURSE OF ANAESTHESIA

Four Stages of Anesthesia

• *Stage of analgesia (from the first effect to unconsciousness):* Increased heart and breathing rates, together with typical pupil dilatation.

- *Stage of excitation (from the beginning of unconsciousness to the start of regular respiration):* Irregular breathing, dilated pupils, heightened motor function, reflexes, nystagmus,
- *Stage of tolerance (from the beginning of regular respiration to the termination of spontaneous respiration):* Small pupils, relaxed skeletal muscles, evident corneal reflex, and absence of eyelid reaction, flat breathing, and effective analgesia.
- *Stage of asphyxia (after termination of the spontaneous diaphragmatic respiration):* Absence of breathing and reflexes poses a risk of mortality, so using antidotes right away is essential to preventing it.

GENERAL ANESTHESIA INDUCTION ROUTES

There are two main approaches to general anesthesia induction.

Injection and Inhalation

- *Injection:* The narcotic chemical dissolves in a liquid when administered *via* this method. IV, IM, SC, or IP may be the administration route. Below is a list of the compounds that are most often used:

- Barbiturates- Phenobarbitone, thiopental-sodium
- Chloral hydrate
- Ketamine
- Hypotonic agents- Mithomidate
- Xylazine
- Urethane

Inhalation: For small laboratory animals like rats, this type of anesthesia is largely ineffective. Larger laboratory animals, including dogs, cats, monkeys, sheep, and goats, are more likely to experience it. The benefits of this anesthetia induction route are the options to precisely regulate the level of anesthetic and the speed at which issues are handled.

PROCEDURE

Rat anesthesia: Xylazine–Ketamine

- Combine 1.25 mL of Xylazine (100 mg/mL) and 8.75 mL of Ketamine (100 mg/mL) in a sterile, 10-milliliter vial with a rubber stopper. Shake well prior to use.
- Keep in a cool, dark area away from light.

- Give 0.05–0.10 mL/100 g intraperitoneally.
- Repeat every thirty minutes or so, using 1/3 to 1/2 doses at a time, as needed.
- Until the animal heals, stop heat loss.

Report: A study was conducted on the impact of general anesthetics in experimental animals.

EUTHANASIA IN EXPERIMENTAL ANIMALS

DESCRIPTION: Killing animals for research is a delicate matter that needs to be handled with extra care to minimize the fear and anguish that the animals experience to the least. The definition of euthanasia is "painless death" in which animals are put to death in labs for the reasons listed below:

- To supply tissues for scientific research when the study is over.
- When there is a chance that the levels of pain, discomfort, or suffering will exceed those set.
- Where there are concerns about the health or well-being of the animals.
- When breeding purposes for animals are no longer served.
- When stock is not needed for certain purposes, such as the use of sex preferences.

GOALS

1. Prevent discomfort and hasten the process of losing consciousness till it happens.
2. Have consistency, repeatability, and irreversibility.
3. Need the least amount of restraint.
4. Take into account the goals of the research.
5. Make administration easy.
6. Make sure the operator is safe.
7. If at all feasible, meet the operator's aesthetic standards.

LOCATION OF EUTHANASIA AND DISPOSAL OF CARCASSES

When killing an animal, it is best to do so in a clean, calm place, away from other animals. Prior to disposing of the corpse, death must be confirmed. Data must be maintained. Tissue from dead animals should, whenever possible, be divided among investigators and instructors. Infants who are dependent on their slain animals must also be destroyed or prepared for their upkeep. Corpses that cannot be disposed of right away must be put on hold.

ANIMALS

Rats, mice, rabbits, and guinea pigs are euthanized by various methods (Table **2**) [2].

Table 2. Methods of euthanasia.

Recommended	Acceptable with Reservations
Chemicals: ***a. Inhalant:*** Isoflurane was used before carbon dioxide. ***b. Injectable:*** Phenobarbitone sodium intraperitoneally.	
Physical: Note that there are no suggested physical techniques.	Cervical dislocation (rats weighing more than 150g should be sedated first) Aesthetically unpleasant decapitation, which may be necessary in certain experimental designs. Aesthetically uncomfortable and stunning exsanguinations

SUGGESTED METHODS FOR CARBON DIOXIDE

An ideal flow rate for carbon dioxide is 20% of the chamber capacity per minute when it is pumped through a reduction valve and into plastic bags or deep containers. Three administration approaches have been the subject of extensive discussion. Carbon dioxide is usedin the following way to put rats and mice to sleep:

- Putting them in a container already filled with carbon dioxide
- Exposing them to air, and then quickly adding carbon dioxide to the container
- Using a mixture of carbon dioxide and oxygen, such as 70% CO_2 and 30% O_2

Phenobarbitone Sodium Injection

Silent induction and death are induced by intraperitoneal administration of phenobarbitone at a dosage of 60 mg/ml at a dose rate of 200 mg/kg. Due to the possibility of residues from the procedure of animal euthanasia, animals or birds should not be given barbiturates.

The high-concentration phenobarbitone solutions for veterinary euthanasia (more than 300 mg/ml) should be diluted with a fast-acting local anesthetic solution since they may cause peritoneal irritation and discomfort.

Strategies that must be used with caution include:

• Cervical dislocation:

In order to do this, the animal must be held prone while the operator applies strong pressure to the neck with the thumb and forefinger, dragging the quarters caudally with the free hand. Although this technique has historically been applied to rats, it may not be visually appealing to the animals; therefore, anesthesia should be given beforehand if this is the case, according to the operator.

• Decapitation:

Despite the common perception that general anesthesia is not aesthetically pleasant, in certain cases, it may be the preferred option for neuroscience research, even though it may interfere with study parameters. In many cases, cervical dislocation is more aesthetically acceptable.

LABORATORY ANIMAL BLOOD COLLECTION TECHNIQUES

PROCEDURE:

Animals: Rat and Mouse.

• Tail Vein Puncture method:
  ○ The animal was confined (Fig. **17**) [3].
  ○ By dipping the tail into water at a 40-to-50-degree angle and rubbing with xylol, the lateral or dorsal veins were dilated. The area was then washed with a disinfectant.
  ○ The thumb and index finger were used to hold onto the tail.
  ○ The 1 ml syringe-equipped 25–27 G needle was inserted close to the distal end of the tail.
  ○ In order to be sure and to prevent the vein wall from collapsing and obliterating the needle aperture, it was sucked.
  ○ Using a sharp object to repeatedly cut the tip of the tail is another method of repeatedly collecting blood.
• Orbital sinus vein puncture:
  ○ Ether was used to anesthetize the animal (Fig. **18**) [4].
  ○ With a gentle twist, the capillary tube was placed in the medial canthus, pointing it caudally and in the direction of the midline.
  ○ After blood collection, pressure was used to avoid hematomas.
  ○ With this technique, 0.5 ml of blood can be drawn once a week.

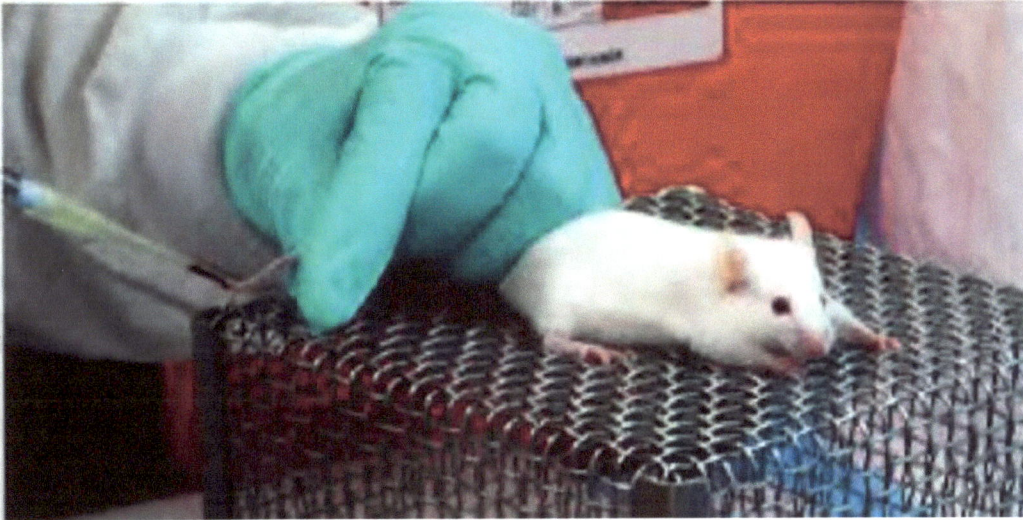

Fig. (17). Tail vein puncture method.

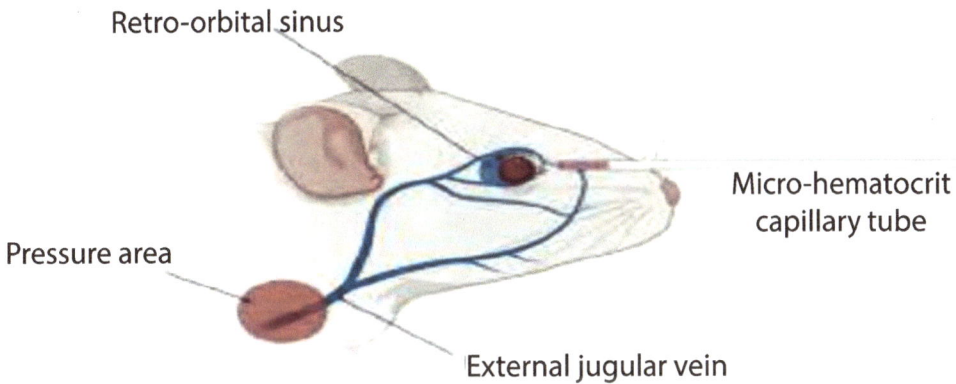

Fig. (18). Orbital sinus vein puncture method.

ANIMAL

Rabbit

Marginal ear vein method:

- A rabbit holder was used to confine the rabbit (Fig. **19**) [5].
- A disinfectant was swabbed, and the lateral edge of the ear was shaved.
- The thumb and index finger were clasped around the ear.
- A 20-G needle was used to pierce the lateral border vein just next to the thumb.
- The vein was aspirated very gently to prevent venous collapse.
- A sample of 0.5–1 ml of blood was taken.

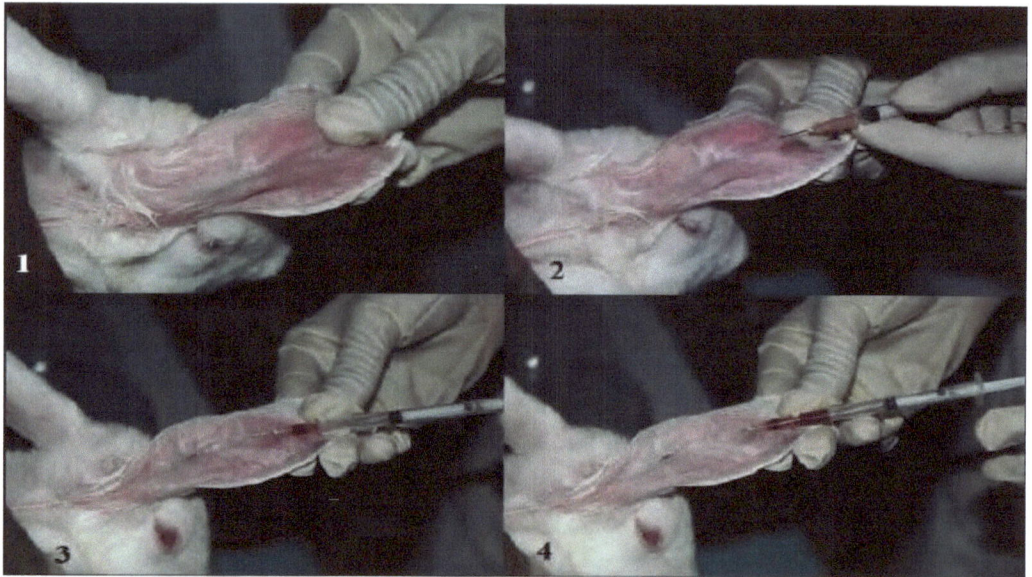

Fig. (19). Marginal ear vein method.

CONCLUSION

The study was able to successfully draw attention to the significance of fundamental laboratory procedures and their subsequent applications. For the purpose of assuring the precision and repeatability of the experiment, skills such as pipetting, weighing, and solution preparation were emphasized as being essential. In the process of assessing and processing biological and chemical materials, advanced techniques such as centrifugation and spectrophotometry have proven their usefulness. It is necessary for a variety of experimental settings to have the capability to precisely monitor pH and to carry out serial dilutions. A robust basis for performing complex experiments in research and industrial contexts can be built *via* the mastery of these procedures. Due to the fact that they have a direct influence on the quality of research results, this experiment highlights the importance of having a strong understanding of typical laboratory techniques. The knowledge that was gathered from this study is extremely significant for students and researchers since it enables them to comprehend and carry out scientific procedures with exceptional accuracy, which guarantees success in future laboratory work.

REFERENCES

[1]   Kelz MB, Mashour GA. The biology of general anesthesia from paramecium to primate. Curr Biol 2019; 29(22): R1199-210.
        [http://dx.doi.org/10.1016/j.cub.2019.09.071] [PMID: 31743680]

[2]   Shomer NH, Allen-Worthington KH, Hickman DL, *et al.* Review of rodent euthanasia methods. J Am

Assoc Lab Anim Sci 2020; 59(3): 242-53.
[http://dx.doi.org/10.30802/AALAS-JAALAS-19-000084] [PMID: 32138808]

[3]   Hu C, Liu H, Lin Z, Liang S, Liu Q, Xu E. A feasible method for vein puncture and drug administration in rats: Ultrasound-guided internal jugular vein puncture. Ultrasound Med Biol. 2025; 51(3): 519-524.
[http://dx.doi.org/10.1016/j.ultrasmedbio.2024.11.013]

[4]   Hoggatt J, Hoggatt AF, Tate TA, Fortman J, Pelus LM. Bleeding the laboratory mouse: Not all methods are equal. Exp Hematol 2016; 44(2): 132-137.e1.
[http://dx.doi.org/10.1016/j.exphem.2015.10.008] [PMID: 26644183]

[5]   Baby PM, Jacob SS, Kumar R, Kumar P. An innovative approach for serial injection in marginal vein and blood collection from auricular artery in New Zealand white Rabbit. MethodsX 2017; 4: 457-60.
[http://dx.doi.org/10.1016/j.mex.2017.11.001] [PMID: 29167756]

CHAPTER 6

Study of Different Routes of Drug Administration in Murines

OBJECTIVE

To study the different routes of drug administration in murine.

PROCEDURE

The following procedures given below are the different routes of drug administration in mice and rats:

Intraperitoneal Injection

- First, the needle's entrance point was found. An imaginary line was drawn above the knees across the abdomen (Fig. **20**) [1].
- A needle was put along the midline, which is on the right side of the animal.
- The point of entry for a female rat or mouse is cranial to the last nostril and slightly medial to it.
- The cecum, a bigger organ on the left side of the abdomen that is packed with fluid, is avoided when the needle is inserted on the right side of the mouse.
- Because the injection might harm the muscle in the back of the leg, it was best to avoid inserting the needle too deeply or laterally from the insertion point. The muscle must be tightly gripped to prevent movement throughout the treatment.
- The mouse needs to be securely confined in order to prevent movement during the IP injection operation.
- The mouse was tilted and constrained such that its abdomen was visible and its head was looking downward. After cleaning the injection site, the needle was placed into the abdomen at a 30-degree angle.
- The needle shaft should be inserted approximately half a centimeter below the surface. To ensure that the needle had not pierced a blood vessel, the intestines, or the bladder, it was aspirated.
- A greenish brown aspirate shows that the needle entered the intestines.
- The process was repeated using a fresh syringe and needle if any fluid was aspirated. The contaminated solution had to be thrown away.

- The injection was administered if no fluid was aspirated. After taking out the needle, the mouse was put back in its cage.
- IP needle size 25–27 G is advised.

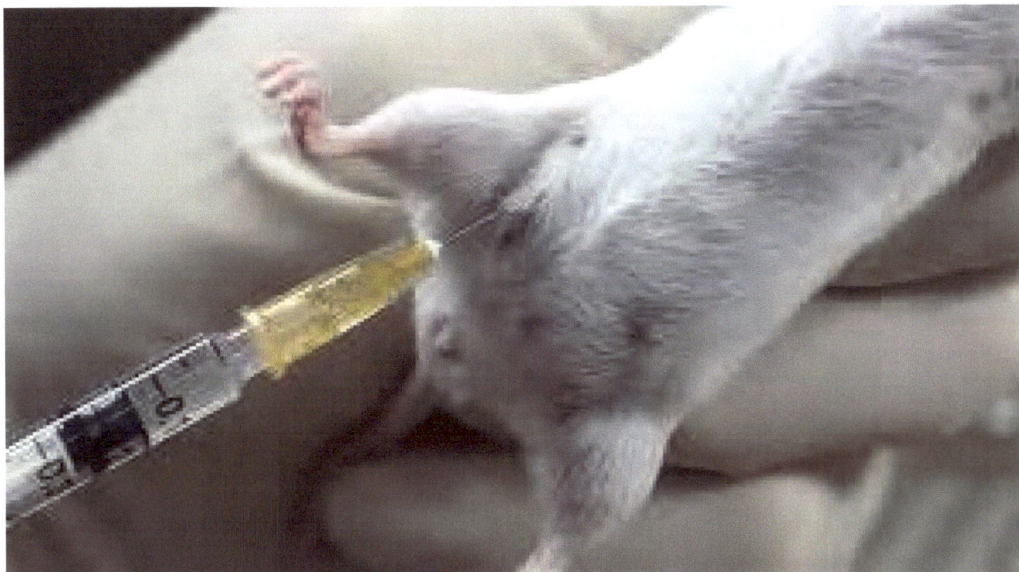

Fig. (20). Intraperitoneal injections.

Precautions for Intraperitoneal Administration in Rats and Mice

Intraperitoneal (IP) administration in rats and mice is a common technique in experimental research, but it requires careful attention to ensure the safety and well-being of the animals. Some key precautions to keep in mind are as follows:

- **Training and Competency:** Only personnel trained and deemed competent in IP injection techniques should perform the procedure.
- **Volume and Concentration:** The volume of the substance injected should be the lowest possible and not exceed the recommended guidelines. For mice, the maximum volume is typically less than 0.5 ml/kg, and for rats, it is less than 2 ml/kg.
- **Needle Size:** Use the appropriate needle size for the species and substance. For mice, a 25-27 gauge needle is recommended, and for rats, a 23-25 gauge needle is suitable.
- **Aseptic Technique:** Maintain aseptic conditions to prevent infection. Use sterile substances, and disinfect the injection site with 70% isopropyl alcohol.
- **Substance Temperature:** Warm the substance to room or body temperature before injection to avoid discomfort and shock.
- **Restraint:** Properly restrain the animal to minimize stress and ensure accurate

injection. For mice, tilt the head slightly downward; for rats, use a gentle but firm hold.
- **Monitoring:** Observe the animals closely after injection for any signs of adverse reactions or complications.

Additional Considerations

- **Frequency of Injections:** Limit the frequency of IP injections to reduce stress and potential complications.
- **Justification:** Provide justification for using IP administration over other routes, as it can be less reliable and more invasive.
- **Ethical Approval:** Ensure all procedures are approved by the relevant animal care and ethics committees.

Subcutaneous Injection

- The skin was raised to create a tent after the mouse was restrained as usual. After cleaning the injection site, the needle was inserted into the subcutaneous tissue (Fig. **21**) [2].
- Before administering the injection, the needle was aspirated; if no aspirate appeared, confirming the correct position, the injection was administered.
- The injection location was chosen to be the area of loose skin around the neck and shoulders.
- Subcutaneous injections were primarily used to inject anesthetics and provide fluids for hydration.
- Average volumes of 1 milliliter or less of the injected area.
- A tent-like structure of folded skin covered the back.
- To prevent puncturing underlying structures, the needle was put at the base of the tent while being held parallel to the animal's body.
- Awoken mice were injected by placing them on the wire lid, allowing them to hang with their front paws during the process. There were scratches on the back skin, and a tent was constructed. A hand was used for scuffing, and a tent was made for both presentation and restraint of the injection site.
- To make sure the needle had not gotten into a blood vessel, it was aspirated.
- The injection rate was modest for the entire volume.
- After removing the needle, the skin was compressed to close the needle's exit hole and stop medication leakage.
- The animal was examined for signs of bleeding.
- A fluid deposit was made in the subcutaneous area, allowing for the visual and tactile perception of the BELB bubble.
- SC needle size 23–25 G is advised.

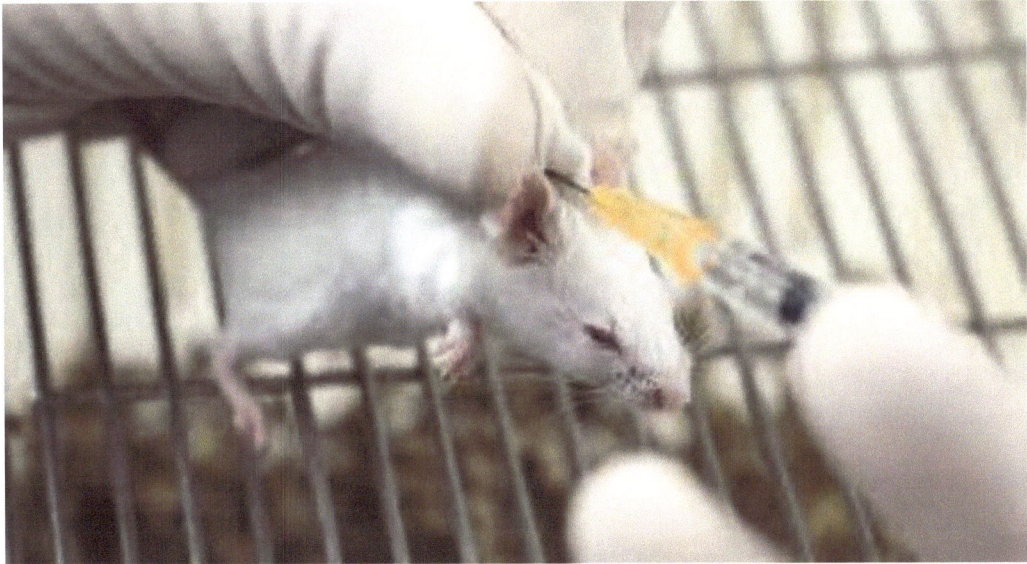

Fig. (21). Subcutaneous injections.

Precautions for S8ubcutaneous Injection

Administering subcutaneous (SC) injections requires careful attention to ensure safety and effectiveness. Here are some key precautions to keep in mind these are as follows:

- **Training and Competency:** Ensure that the person administering the injection is properly trained and competent in SC injection techniques.
- **Needle Size and Type:** Use the appropriate needle size and type for the medication and the patient's body type. Typically, a 25–27-gauge needle is used for SC injections.
- **Injection Site Selection:** Common sites for SC injections include the abdomen, the upper arm, and the thigh. Rotate injection sites to prevent tissue damage and ensure proper absorption.
- **Aseptic Technique:** Maintain aseptic conditions to prevent infection. Clean the injection site with an alcohol swab and use sterile needles and syringes.
- **Volume and Injection Angle:** The volume of medication should be appropriate for SC administration, usually not exceeding 1 ml. Inject at a 45 to 90-degree angle, depending on the amount of subcutaneous tissue.
- **Do Not Aspirate:** Unlike intramuscular injections, do not aspirate (pull back on the syringe) before injecting the medication.
- **Monitor for Reactions:** Observe the injection site for any signs of adverse reactions, such as redness, swelling, or pain. Report any unusual symptoms to a healthcare provider.

- **Patient Comfort:** Ensure the patient is comfortable and relaxed during the injection process to minimize discomfort and anxiety.

Additional Considerations

- **Frequency of Injections:** Limit the frequency of injections to avoid tissue damage and discomfort.
- **Proper Disposal:** Dispose of used needles and syringes in a sharps container to prevent needle-stick injuries.
- **Patient Education:** Educate patients on how to self-administer SC injections if necessary, including proper technique and site rotation.
- **Awareness:**Be aware of the availability of the injections and provide the specified awareness of the administrative generals.

Intramuscular Injection

- Since mice have little muscle mass, intramuscular injections are not advised.
- An injection might hurt and irritate nearby tissues (Fig. **22**) [3].

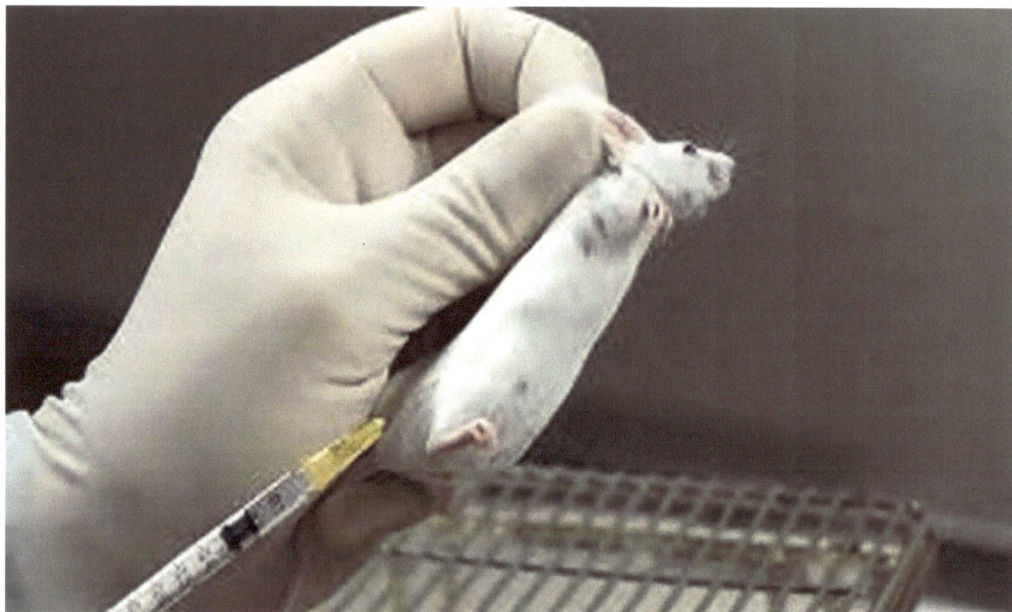

Fig. (22). Intramuscular injections.

Precautions for Intramuscular Administration

The key precautions to consider for intramuscular (IM) administration to ensure safety and effectiveness:

- **Training and Competency:** Ensure that the person administering the injection is properly trained and competent in IM injection techniques.
- **Needle Size and Length:** Choose the appropriate needle size and length based on the patient's age, muscle mass, and the type of medication. Typically, a 22–25-gauge needle is used, with a length of 1 to 1.5 inches.
- **Injection Sites:** Common sites for IM injections include the deltoid muscle of the upper arm, the vastus lateralis muscle of the thigh, and the ventrogluteal and dorsogluteal muscles of the buttocks. Rotate injection sites to prevent tissue damage and ensure proper absorption.
- **Aseptic Technique:** Maintain aseptic conditions to prevent infection. Clean the injection site with an alcohol swab and use sterile needles and syringes.
- **Volume and Injection Angle:** The volume of medication should be appropriate for IM administration, usually not exceeding 2-5 ml, depending on the site and the patient. Inject at a 90-degree angle to the skin.
- **Aspiration:** After inserting the needle, aspirate (pull back on the syringe) to check for blood. If blood appears, choose a new site to avoid injecting into a blood vessel.
- **Patient Comfort:** Ensure the patient is comfortable and relaxed during the injection process to minimize discomfort and anxiety. Use a quick, smooth motion to insert the needle.
- **Monitor for Reactions:** Observe the injection site for any signs of adverse reactions, such as redness, swelling, or pain. Report any unusual symptoms to a healthcare provider.

Additional Considerations

- **Frequency of Injections:** Limit the frequency of injections to avoid tissue damage and discomfort.
- **Proper Disposal:** Dispose of used needles and syringes in a sharps container to prevent needle-stick injuries.
- **Patient Education:** Educate patients on how to manage potential side effects and care for the injection site if they receive frequent IM injections.

Intravenous Injection

- The mouse's tail vein was utilized.
- The mouse's tail vein was utilized; chemical or physical restraint was used to confine the mouse. To see the vein, the tail was slightly twisted.
- After cleaning the injection site and inserting a 27–30 G needle slowly into the vein—not allowing for aspiration—the injection was administered while the lumen was being monitored for cleanliness.

- A little bulge in the tail was the result of incorrect placement; the procedure was repeated close to the original spot after the needle was removed, and pressure was then applied at the injection site (Fig. **23**) [4].

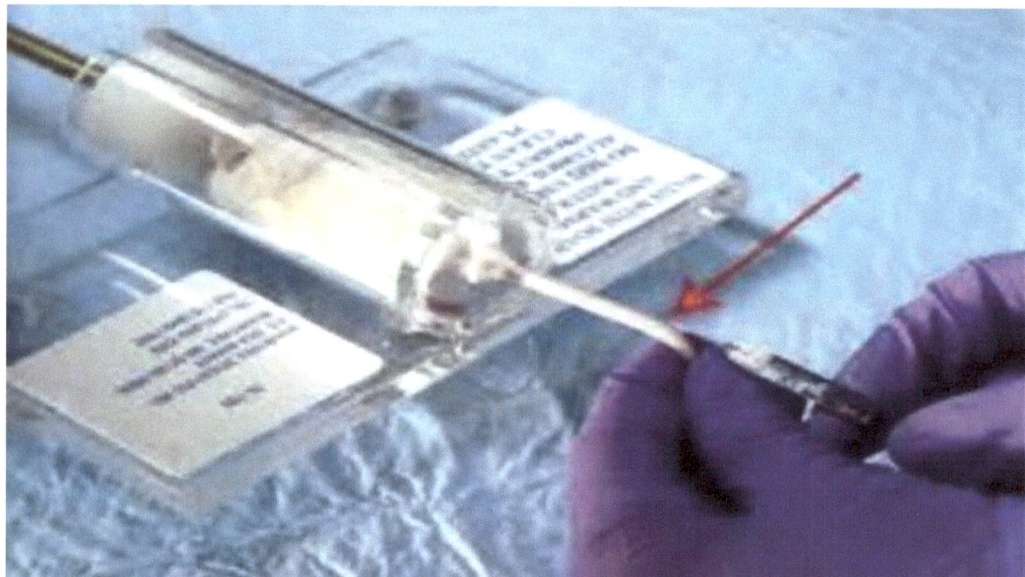

Fig. (23). Intravenous injection.

Precautions for Intravenous Injection

Intravenous (IV) injections are a common method for administering medications and fluids directly into the bloodstream. However, they require strict adherence to safety protocols to prevent complications. Some key precautions to consider for IV administration are as follows:

- **Training and Competency:** Ensure that the person administering the IV injection is properly trained and competent in IV techniques.
- **Sterile Technique:** Maintain aseptic conditions to prevent infections. Use sterile gloves, needles, syringes, and disinfect the injection site with an alcohol swab.
- **Vein Selection:** Choose an appropriate vein, typically in the arm or hand. Avoid veins that are swollen, hardened, or previously damaged.
- **Needle and Catheter Size:** Select the appropriate needle or catheter size based on the patient's vein size and the type of medication. A 20- 25-gauge needle is commonly used for adults.
- **Injection Site Preparation:** Clean the injection site thoroughly with an antiseptic solution to reduce the risk of infection.
- **Proper Insertion Technique:** Insert the needle or catheter at a low angle to the skin, typically 15-30 degrees, to ensure it enters the vein without causing

trauma.
- **Monitor for Complications:** Watch for signs of complications such as infiltration (fluid leaking into surrounding tissue), phlebitis (vein inflammation), or infection. Stop the infusion immediately if complications arise.
- **Slow Administration:** Administer the medication slowly to avoid adverse reactions, especially with certain drugs that can cause severe reactions if given too quickly.
- **Patient Monitoring:** Monitor the patient closely for any signs of adverse reactions, such as pain, swelling, or allergic reactions. Be prepared to respond to emergencies.

Additional Considerations

- **Volume and Rate of Infusion:** Ensure the volume and rate of infusion are appropriate for the patient's condition and the type of medication being administered.
- **Proper Disposal:** Dispose of used needles and syringes in a sharps container to prevent needle-stick injuries.
- **Patient Education:** Educate patients on what to expect during and after the IV injection, including potential side effects and how to care for the injection site.

Intradermal Injection

- Only under anesthesia was the intradermal injection performed.
- The back hair was trimmed and prepped with an alcohol swab.
- On the back, a 30-degree angle was used to place the needle between the skin layers.
- In order to guarantee correct implantation, the syringe was aspirated.
- Any blood or other fluid-related signs suggested incorrect installation.
- To prevent tissue stress, the medication was injected slowly, with a maximum amount of 100µl at the injection site. A tiny circular melt was produced by a successful injection (Fig. **24**) [5].

Precautions for Intradermal Injections

Administering intradermal (ID) injections requires precision and care to ensure safety and effectiveness. Here are some key precautions to keep in mind:

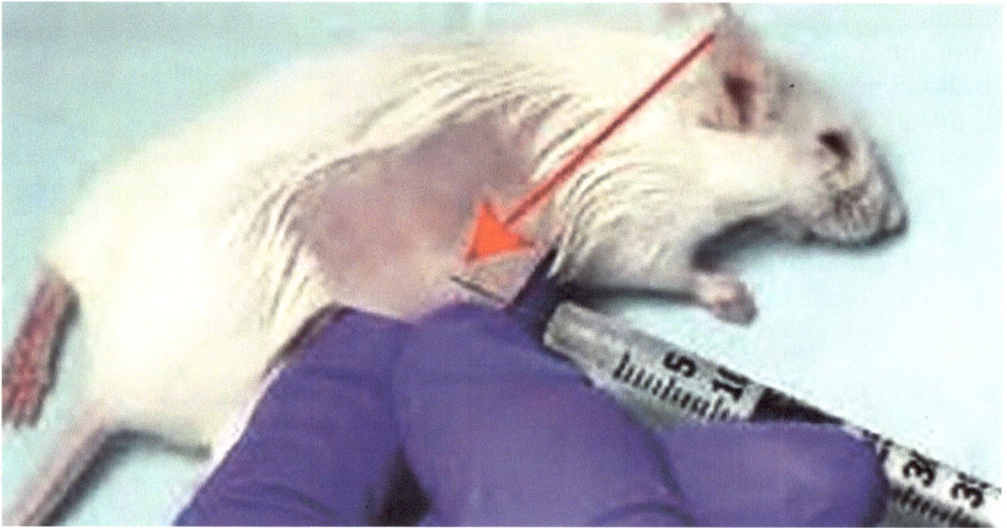

Fig. (24). Intradermal injection.

Precautions for Intradermal Injection

- **Training and Competency:** Ensure that the person administering the injection is properly trained and competent in ID injection techniques.
- **Needle Size and Type:** Use a short, fine needle, typically 26-27 gauge, 3/8 to 1/2 inch in length, appropriate for intradermal injections.
- **Injection Sites:** Common sites for ID injections include the inner forearm and upper back, where the skin is relatively thin and easy to access.
- **Aseptic Technique:** Maintain aseptic conditions to prevent infections. Clean the injection site with an alcohol swab and use sterile needles and syringes.
- **Proper Injection Angle:** Insert the needle at a shallow angle, usually 5 to 15 degrees, with the bevel facing up. Ensure that the needle enters just into the dermis, creating a small raised bleb or wheal.
- **Volume of Injection:** The volume of medication should be small, usually 0.1 ml to 0.2 ml, to prevent tissue damage and ensure proper absorption.
- **Do Not Aspirate:** Unlike intramuscular injections, do not aspirate (pull back on the syringe) before injecting the medication.
- **Monitor for Reactions:** Observe the injection site for any signs of adverse reactions, such as redness, swelling, or pain. Report any unusual symptoms to a healthcare provider.
- **Patient Comfort:** Ensure the patient is comfortable and relaxed during the injection process to minimize discomfort and anxiety.

Additional Considerations

- **Proper Disposal:** Dispose of used needles and syringes in a sharps container to prevent needle-stick injuries.
- **Patient Education:** Educate patients on what to expect during and after the ID injection, including potential side effects and how to care for the injection site.
- **Documentation:** Record the details of the injection, including the site, volume, and any observed reactions, for proper medical records.

Oral Route

- A 1-3 ml syringe was used with biomedical needles.
- The measurement was taken from the tip of the nose to the first rib. A measured-length needle was utilized.
- The right amount of medication was put into the syringe.
- The mouse was under a restraint.
- The tip slipped along the back of the mouth, pushing the lip forward with a single, felt action.
- Anything felt suggested an incorrect placement.
- After the needle was inserted correctly, the medication was given (Fig. **25**) [6].

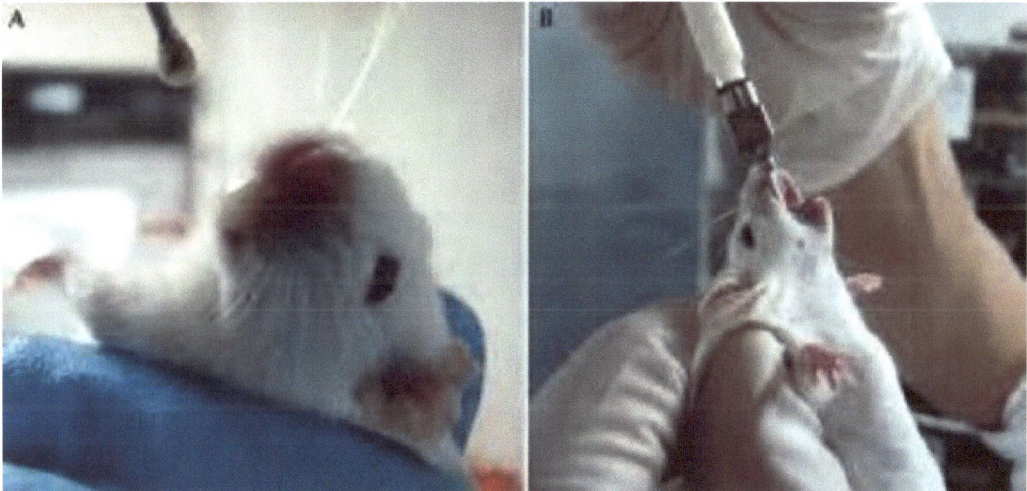

Fig. (25). Oral Route.

Precautions for Oral Route Administration

Oral route administration is one of the most common and convenient methods of delivering medications. However, it still requires specific precautions to ensure safety and effectiveness. Here are some key considerations:

Precautions for Oral Route Administration

- **Proper Dosage:** Ensure that the prescribed dosage is accurate and appropriate for the patient. Double-check the medication label and dosage instructions.
- **Timing:** Administer the medication at the correct time intervals, as prescribed. Some medications must be taken with food, while others should be taken on an empty stomach.
- **Patient Position:** Encourage the patient to sit or stand upright when taking the medication to prevent choking and ensure proper swallowing.
- **Swallowing Difficulties:** Be aware of any swallowing difficulties the patient may have. For patients with dysphagia, consider alternatives such as liquid formulations or consult a healthcare provider for advice.
- **Crushing or Splitting Tablets:** Only crush or split tablets if it is safe to do so and if it does not affect the medication's efficacy. Some medications are designed for slow release and should not be altered.
- **Interaction with Food and Drink:** Be aware of potential interactions with certain foods, beverages, or other medications. For example, grapefruit juice can interfere with the metabolism of some drugs.
- **Hydration:** Ensure the patient drinks sufficient water with the medication to aid swallowing and absorption.
- **Allergies and Sensitivities:** Check for any known allergies or sensitivities to the medication or its components.
- **Storage:** Store medications properly, according to the manufacturer's instructions, to maintain their potency and safety.
- **Education:** Educate the patient on the importance of adherence to the medication regimen and how to take the medication correctly.

Additional Considerations

- **Monitoring:** Observe the patient for any adverse reactions or side effects and report them to a healthcare provider immediately.
- **Documentation:** Record the administration details, including the time, dosage, and any observations, to ensure accurate medical records.
- **Missed Doses:** Provide instructions on what to do if a dose is missed, including whether to take it as soon as one remembers or to skip it if it is close to the next scheduled dose.

CONCLUSION

It was established through the experiment that the route of drug administration has a substantial impact on the pharmacological effects, absorption, and bioavailability of medicines in mice and rats. Because of first-pass metabolism, oral delivery was slower than intravenous administration, which resulted in the earliest onset of action and maximum efficacy. Intravenous administration was the most effective method. Intermediate effects were produced by both intraperitoneal and subcutaneous administration, which were influenced by the solubility and the local absorption of the drug. These findings highlight how important it is to choose the optimal route of administration based on the therapeutic requirements and the characteristics of the medicine. As a result of this study, the utilization of animal models for the purpose of comprehending drug kinetics and dynamics is validated, which contributes to the optimization of drug delivery systems. In addition to this, it lays the groundwork for the interpretation of preclinical findings into clinical applications, which guarantees the efficient and risk-free utilization of pharmaceuticals in a variety of therapeutic environments.

REFERENCES

[1]   Practical Antimicrobial Therapeutics. In: Veterinary Medicine. Elsevier; 2017. p. 153–74.
        [http://dx.doi.org/10.1016/B978-0-7020-5246-0.00006-1]

[2]   Mathias N, Huille S, Picci M, *et al.* Towards more tolerable subcutaneous administration: Review of contributing factors for improving combination product design. Adv Drug Deliv Rev 2024; 209: 115301.
        [http://dx.doi.org/10.1016/j.addr.2024.115301] [PMID: 38570141]

[3]   Nicoll LH, Hesby A. Intramuscular injection: An integrative research review and guideline for evidence-based practice. Appl Nurs Res 2002; 15(3): 149-62.
        [http://dx.doi.org/10.1053/apnr.2002.34142] [PMID: 12173166]

[4]   Wagner M, Koester H, Deffge C, Weinert S, Lauf J, Francke A, *et al.* Isolation and intravenous injection of murine bone marrow derived monocytes. Journal of Visualized Experiments. 2014 Dec 27; (94).

[5]   Moser HR, Giesler GJ Jr. Itch elicited by intradermal injection of serotonin, intracisternal injection of morphine, and their synergistic interactions in rats. Neuroscience 2014; 274: 119-27.
        [http://dx.doi.org/10.1016/j.neuroscience.2014.05.025] [PMID: 24875173]

[6]   Nebendahl K. Routes of Administration. The Laboratory Rat. Elsevier 2000; pp. 463-83.
        [http://dx.doi.org/10.1016/B978-012426400-7.50063-7]

Effects of Hepatic Microsomal Enzyme Inducers on Phenobarbitone-Induced Sleep Duration in Mice

OBJECTIVE

Study the effect of hepatic microsomal enzyme inducers on the phenobarbitone-induced sleeping time in mice.

REQUIREMENTS

Animals: Mice.

Drugs: Phenobarbitone sodium (dose: 50mg/kg IP), Pentobarbital sodium (dose: 45 mg/kg IP).

Microsomal Enzyme Inducers and Their Types

Microsomal enzyme inducers are substances that enhance the activity and expression of microsomal enzymes, particularly those of the **cytochrome P450 (CYP)** enzyme family, in the liver and other tissues. These enzymes are crucial for the metabolism of drugs, endogenous compounds (*e.g.*, steroids), and xenobiotics [1].

Types of Microsomal Enzyme Inducers

Microsomal enzyme inducers can be broadly categorized based on their chemical nature or the specific enzymes they induce [2].

Pharmacological Inducers

These are drugs that enhance the activity of microsomal enzymes:

- **Rifampin:** A potent inducer of CYP3A4 and other enzymes.
- **Carbamazepine:** Induces CYP3A4, CYP1A2, and CYP2C9.
- **Phenytoin:** Induces CYP3A4, CYP2C9, and CYP2C19.
- **Phenobarbital:** Induces a wide range of CYP enzymes.
- **Dexamethasone:** Induces CYP3A4 and CYP2C enzymes.

Dietary and Herbal Inducers

- **St. John's Wort:** Induces CYP3A4 and P-glycoprotein, affecting drug bioavailability.
- **Cruciferous Vegetables (*e.g.*, broccoli, cabbage):** Contain indoles that induce CYP1A enzymes.
- **Grapefruit:**Induces paradoxical effect depending on compounds.

Environmental Inducers

- **Polycyclic Aromatic Hydrocarbons (PAHs):** Found in tobacco smoke and charred meat; they induce CYP1A enzymes.
- **Pesticides and Herbicides:** Induce enzymes involved in xenobiotic metabolism.

Endogenous Compounds

- Certain **hormones** or physiological states can lead to enzyme induction. For example, **glucocorticoids**, which induce CYP3A enzymes.

Synthetic and Industrial Chemical

Alcohol: Chronic alcohol consumption induces CYP2E1, which metabolizes ethanol and other toxins.

CLINICAL IMPLICATIONS OF ENZYME INDUCTION

1. **Altered Drug Metabolism:**
   - Enhanced metabolism may reduce drug efficacy (*e.g.*, oral contraceptives).
   - Increased formation of toxic metabolites in some cases (*e.g.*, acetaminophen and CYP2E1).
2. **Drug Interactions:**
   - Concurrent use of enzyme inducers with other medications may necessitate dose adjustments.
3. **Disease Impact:**
   - Conditions like porphyria can worsen due to increased heme synthesis.
4. **Environmental Exposures:**
   - Prolonged exposure to environmental inducers (*e.g.*, smoking) affects the metabolism of many drugs [3].

PRINCIPLE

Substances that activate the hepatic microsomal oxidative enzyme system improve how well other substances are metabolized. Consequently, the duration of the effect of the second medicine will be diminished in the presence of an enzyme inducer. This has important therapeutic implications because when multiple medications are given concurrently, one medication may induce the activity of microsomal enzymes and one can alter the activity of another. Typical medications that trigger the hepatic microsomal enzyme system include Meprobamate with phenobarbitone. Any medication administered in combination with any of these medications may have an impact on how the second drug is disposed of, and thus, the intended pharmaceutical outcomes.

PROCEDURE

• Weigh and number the animals. Split them up into two groups of no fewer than six mice each.
• Give the first group one injection of phenobarbitone every day for five days. Give the other group the same distilled water for five days.
• On the fifth day, inject Phenobarbital into both groups one hour after the previous dosage of phenobarbitone.
• Observe how long the phenobarbitone-induced sleep lasted in each group and when it started.

INFERENCE: In contrast to animals that received distilled water treatment, animals pretreated with phenobarbitone slept for shorter periods of time.

REPORT: A study was conducted on the impact of hepatic microsomal inducers on the sleeping period of mice treated with phenobarbitone.

CONCLUSION

The results of the experiment demonstrated that hepatic microsomal enzyme inducers considerably cut down on the amount of time that mice spent sleeping as a result of phenobarbitone. This finding lends credence to the hypothesis that enzyme induction speeds up the metabolism of the drug. The hepatic enzyme activity was increased by pre-treatment with medicines such as phenobarbital and rifampicin, which resulted in a quicker clearance of phenobarbitone from the system and a shorter duration of drowsiness. In addition to shedding light on the significance of hepatic microsomal enzymes in the process of drug metabolism, these findings offer valuable insights that can be utilized to better comprehend the interactions between drugs, particularly in the context of enzyme enhancement. The study highlights the possibility of altered pharmacological efficacy due to changes in drug metabolism, which has substantial implications for clinical pharmacology. These implications are especially relevant when it comes to the management of patients who are undergoing long-term therapy with enzyme inducers and barbiturates.

REFERENCES

[1]   Kato R, Chiesara E, Vassanelli P. Factors influencing induction of hepatic microsomal drug-metabolizing enzymes. Biochem Pharmacol 1962; 11(3): 211-20.
[http://dx.doi.org/10.1016/0006-2952(62)90076-X] [PMID: 14454283]

[2]   Ioannides C, Parke DV. Mechanism of induction of hepatic microsomal drug metabolizing enzymes by a series of barbiturates. J Pharm Pharmacol 1975; 27(10): 739-46.
[http://dx.doi.org/10.1111/j.2042-7158.1975.tb09393.x] [PMID: 241786]

[3]   Doo Kim N, Keun Yoo J, Me Won S, Shin Park S, Gelboin HV. Phenytoin induction of cytochrome P4502B in mice: effects on hexobarbital hydroxylase activity. Xenobiotica 1993; 23(3): 217-25.
[http://dx.doi.org/10.3109/00498259309059376] [PMID: 8498085]

CHAPTER 8

Drugs Acting on Ciliary Motility of Frog Esophagus

OBJECTIVE

To study the effects of drugs on the ciliary motility of the frog esophagus using the ExPharm T2 version.

PRINCIPLE

Cilia are found in the frog esophagus. The function of acetylcholine in the mucous membrane is necessary for ciliary motion. ACh stimulates cilia to contract, which increases movement. Anti-cholinergic medications immobilize cilia and have comparable effects to cholinergic medicines, which lessen their motion. To illustrate, this experiment uses a handful of these medications to obtain their result [1].

REQUIREMENTS

1. Frog
2. Poppy seeds
3. Frog board
4. Stop watch

Drugs and Solutions

a. Frog ringer (NaCl 8g/L, KCl 0.2g/L, CaCl$_2$ 0.1g/L , MgSO$_4$ 0.1g/L)
b. Physostigmine 10%
c. Atropine 0.1%
d. Acetylcholine 10%

SET UP: A frog's lower jaw is extracted together with its pith. An opening is made in the esophagus from the buccal cavity to the stomach. It iseverted and pinned onto a wooden board. Blood is eliminated from frogs by using a cotton swab soaked in Ringer's solution. The surface is dampened with Ringer's solution, and a poppy seed is positioned at the head's end. In the esophagus, motions and the amount of time needed to traverse a certain distance are noted (Fig. **26**) [2].

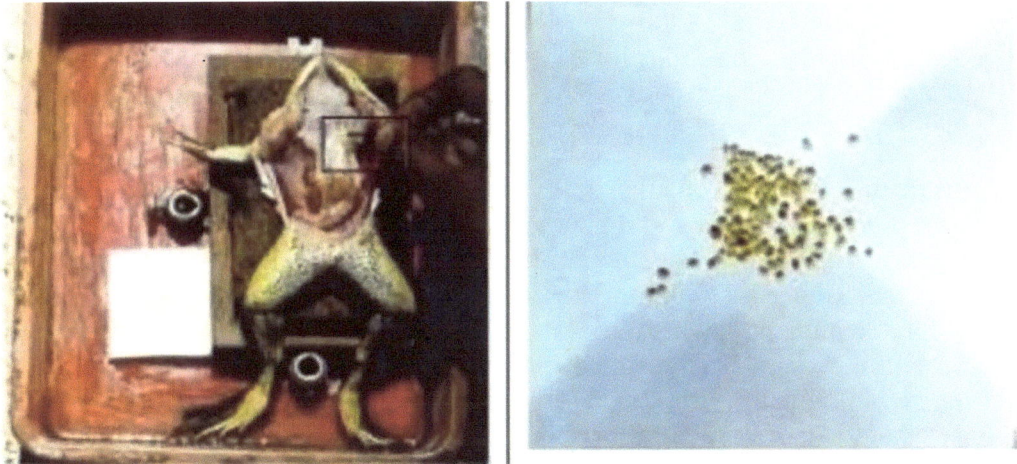

Fig. (26). A Poppy seed being placed in the esophagus.

PROCEDURE

1. Calculate the seed's migration distance. Pins positioned at the caudal (distal) end and the cephalic end, respectively, will serve as the beginning and ending points.
2. Apply Ringer's solutionto the esophageal surface. At the cephalic end of the esophagus, plant a poppy seed. Because of ciliary motility, the seed begins to move. Start the stopwatch when the seed passes the cephalic end pins, which serve as the beginning point. When the seed reaches the distal pins, stop the watch.
3. Record how long it takes for the seed to cover the distance. To receive three readings, repeat step two again.
4. Take three readings after administering ACh.
5. Carry out steps two and three again.
6. Take three readings after administering physostigmine.
7. Carry out steps two and three again.
8. Take three readings after administering atropine.
9. After step 6, instill ACh and see its impact (without utilizing frog-Ringer). Compare it to the result achieved using ACh alone (Step 4).
10. Write conclusions after tabulating your readings.

NOTE

1. Determine the average reading for each drug after testing it three times, including that for Ringer's solution.
2. Readings for Ringer's solution are used as a control and contrasted with test (drug) readings.
3. Prior to testing any drug, obtain readings using Ringer's solution and take

separate control readings for each substance.

4. Use new preparations (frog) for each drug. Drugs should be applied to the same preparation (frog) consecutively without using Ringer's solution in between in order to observe interactions.

To ensure accurate and reliable results when testing the effects of different drugs using frog preparations, a systematic approach is essential. Firstly, for each drug, the average reading should be determined after conducting three tests, including that for the Ringer's solution. The readings for Ringer's solution serve as a control and compared against the test readings for each drug. Before testing any drug, control readings using the Ringer's solution must be obtained for each substance individually. It is crucial to use a new frog preparation for each drug. Drugs should be applied consecutively to the same preparation without interspersing with Ringer's solution in between to observe any potential interactions between the drugs. This method allows for accurate comparisons and the observation of drug interactions, ensuring the reliability and validity of the experimental results.

OBSERVATION

REPORT

A study was conducted to study the effects of drugs on the ciliary motility of frog esophagus (Table **3**) using Expharm T2 version.

Table 3. Effect of drugs on the ciliary motility of frog esophagus [3].

S.No.	Drugs	Reading 1	Reading 2	Reading 3	Mean
1.	Ringer	-	-	-	-
2.	Acetylcholine	-	-	-	-
3.	Physostigmine	-	-	-	-
4.	Atropine	-	-	-	-

CONCLUSION

During the course of the experiment, it was successfully established that different medicines have different effects on the ciliary motility of the esophagus of the animal. It is clear that acetylcholine has a function in promoting ciliary activity through cholinergic pathways because it was found to enhance the frequency of ciliary beats. The effects of adrenaline were contradictory, which suggests that it has a complex relationship with adrenergic receptors. On the other hand, local anesthetics such as procaine decrease ciliary motility, most likely because of the membrane-stabilizing qualities that they possess. The pharmacological modulation of ciliary motility, which is an essential component of mucosal defense mechanisms, is better understood as a result of these results, which will lead to a better understanding of the topic. The findings also emphasize the potential of employing frog esophagus models for the purpose of researching the effects of drugs on ciliary function. This could be useful for the development of therapeutic medicines that target problems related to mucociliary clearance.

REFERENCES

[1]   Hill JR. The influence of drugs on ciliary activity. J Physiol 1957; 139(2): 157-66.
[http://dx.doi.org/10.1113/jphysiol.1957.sp005883] [PMID: 13492205]

[2]   Hughes J. Isolation of an endogenous compound from the brain with pharmacological properties similar to morphine. Brain Res 1975; 88(2): 295-308.
[http://dx.doi.org/10.1016/0006-8993(75)90391-1] [PMID: 1148827]

[3]   Slaughter M, Aiello E. Cholinergic nerves stimulate mucociliary transport, ciliary activity, and mucus secretion in the frog palate. Cell Tissue Res 1982; 227(2): 413-21.
[http://dx.doi.org/10.1007/BF00210895] [PMID: 6983908]

CHAPTER 9

Impact of Several Drugs on the Rabbit Eye

OBJECTIVE

To study the effect of drugs on the rabbit eye.

PRINCIPLE

Many medications are applied topically as ointments or drops to target specific areas of the eye. The majority of these medications fall into the autonomic, local anesthetic, or antimicrobial pharmacological classes. Nerves that supply the eye are both sympathetic and parasympathetic. The dilator papillae of the iris and the superior palpebral muscle are supplied sympathetically. The parasympathetic nervous system controls the sphincter pupillae of the iris. Furthermore, as the parasympathetic nerve contracts, the ciliary muscle flexes inward and forward, receiving its supply from the ciliary body. The eye is adapted for close vision because of the forward protrusion of the lens. On the other hand, the paralysis of the accommodation process is brought about by the relaxation of the ciliary muscle. Drugs given topically can alter the cornea's sensitivity, light reflex, intraocular pressure, conjunctival congestion, and papillary size. Nonetheless, students may readily research how drugs affect corneal reflex, light reflex, and papillary size. A clear plastic scale can be used to measure the eye's pupil size by positioning it in front of the eye as close as feasible. A torch's light pointed at the pupil will cause a light reflex. A sterile thin cotton swab is used to gently contact the cornea from the side so that the patient does not see it. This causes a corneal reflex, which causes the crystals to blink.

A mydriatic is a type of medication that causes the pupil of the eye to dilate (widen). Mydriatics are often used during eye examinations to allow the ophthalmologist or optometrist to get a better view of the inside of the eye, including the retina and optic nerve. These medications can also be used in the treatment of certain eye conditions, such as uveitis, where dilating the pupil can help alleviate pain and prevent the formation of adhesions within the eye.

Common mydriatic agents include:

- **Atropine**
- **Tropicamide**
- **Phenylephrine**

Miosis:

Miosis refers to the constriction of the pupil of the eye. It occurs when the muscles in the iris contract, making the pupil smaller. Miosis can be a normal physiological response to bright light, as the eye adjusts to protect the retina from excessive light exposure. It can also be induced by certain medications, such as miotic drugs, or occur due to various medical conditions.

Common causes of miosis include:

- **Exposure to bright light**
- **Certain medications** (*e.g.*, pilocarpine)
- **Opioid use**
- **Neurological conditions**
- **Eye injuries**

REQUIREMENTS

Animal: Rabbit (2-5kg); Drugs: Atropine (1%w/v) and Physostigmine (1%w/v)

EQUIPMENT

rabbit holder, pen torch

PROCEDURE

1. Keeping the head outside, place the rabbit in the rabbit holder.
2. Examine the size of the pupils in each eye.
3. Hold the torch in front of the rabbit's eyes and move the light beam to see the effects of light reflex.
4. Examine the corneal reflex by using a cotton swab to touch the cornea.
5. As a control, inject a few drops of atropine solution into the rabbit's right eye's conjunctiva over the course of eight to ten minutes. Fill the left eye with regular saline.
6. After the drug has been initialized for ten minutes, measure the pupil size, light reflex, and corneal reflex, then tabulate the results.
7. Conduct the same trials using ephedrine and physostigmine.

Table 4. Effect of Different Drugs on Pupillary Size, Light Reflex, and Corneal Reflex.

Drug	Pupillary Size	Light reflex	Corneal reflex
Saline	Normal	Present	Present
Physostigmine	Constriction	Present	Present
Ephedrine	Dilation	Present	Present
Atropine	Dilation	Absent	Present

INFERENCE

Saline: Instilling saline has no effect on pupil size. Light reflexes are present.

Physostigmine: Reduces iris diameter and pupil size, resulting in miosis. Reflexes to light and touch are present.

Ephedrine: Propecia enlarges the pupil and dilates the iris, resulting in mydriasis. The light reflex is still lacking, but the touch reflex and light reflex are present.

Atropine: Increases the pupil size and the diameter of the iris, thereby causing mydriasis.

While there is a touch reflex, there is no light reflex. Table **4** is followed by the reference [1].

CONCLUSION

The experiment successfully illustrated the impacts of different medications on the ocular functions of rabbits, shedding light on the roles of atropine, pilocarpine, and tetracaine in ocular pharmacology. Atropine, a mydriatic, causes pupil dilation, while pilocarpine, a miotic, induces pupil constriction. Tetracaine, an anesthetic, effectively blocks reflex reactions. These findings are significant because they underscore the utility of rabbits in ocular drug testing, providing valuable insights into the pharmacological effects of topical medicines used in ophthalmology [2].

The study highlights several important aspects:

1. **Atropine**: This drug is responsible for the dilation of pupils. In ophthalmology, this property is particularly useful for eye examinations and surgeries, allowing better visualization of the eye's internal structures [3].
2. **Pilocarpine**: Known for its ability to constrict the pupils, pilocarpine is essential in treating conditions such as glaucoma. Reducing the pupil size helps

decrease intraocular pressure, which is crucial in managing glaucoma.

3. **Tetracaine**: As an anesthetic, tetracaine blocks reflex activity, making it invaluable during eye surgeries and procedures. It ensures that the patient does not experience pain or discomfort during the process [4].

REFERENCES

[1]   Ahn SJ, Hong HK, Na YM, Park SJ, Ahn J, Oh J, *et al*. Use of rabbit eyes in pharmacokinetic studies of intraocular drugs. Journal of Visualized Experiments. 2016 Jul 23; (113).

[2]   Fernandez V, Fragoso MA, Billotte C, *et al*. Efficacy of various drugs in the prevention of posterior capsule opacification: Experimental study of rabbit eyes. J Cataract Refract Surg 2004; 30(12): 2598-605.
       [http://dx.doi.org/10.1016/j.jcrs.2004.05.013] [PMID: 15617931]

[3]   Chiou GCY, Yan HY. Effects of antiglaucoma drugs on the blood flow in rabbit eyes. Ophthalmic Res 1986; 18(5): 265-9.
       [http://dx.doi.org/10.1159/000265445] [PMID: 3808590]

[4]   Ahn SJ, Hong HK, Na YM, Park SJ, Ahn J, Oh J, et al. Use of Rabbit Eyes in Pharmacokinetic Studies of Intraocular Drugs. Journal of Visualized Experiments. 2016 Jul 23; (113).

CHAPTER 10

Impact of Skeletal Muscle Relaxants Assessed *via* Rotarod Apparatus

OBJECTIVE

To study the effect of skeletal muscle relaxants using the Rotarod apparatus.

PRINCIPLE

Muscle relaxing ability is one of the key pharmacological actions of anti-anxiety medications in the benzodiazepine class of pharmaceuticals. These substances have a calming or sedative effect, in addition to relaxing skeletal muscles, which helps lower tension and anxiety. One sign of muscle relaxation is a loss of grip. Easily tested on animals, this effect can be measured with an inclined plane or revolving rods. An indicator of muscle relaxation is the difference in the fall-off time of the rotating rod between the animal in the diazepam-treated group and the animal in the control group. It is necessary to adjust the inclined plane's slope angle or the rod's spinning speed so that an average mouse can stay on the plane or on the rod for a significant period of time.

Skeletal Muscle Relaxant

A skeletal muscle relaxant is a type of medication that affects skeletal muscle function and decreases muscle tone. These drugs are used to alleviate symptoms such as muscle spasms, pain, and hyperreflexia [1]. There are two main types of muscle relaxants:

Neuromuscular blockers: These act by interfering with transmission at the neuromuscular end plate and are often used during surgical procedures to cause temporary paralysis.

1. **Spasmolytics (centrally acting muscle relaxants)**: These work within the central nervous system to alleviate musculoskeletal pain and spasms.

REQUIREMENT

Animal: Mice weighing 20–25 grams

Drugs: Administer 1 milliliter per 100 grams of the mouse's body weight using a diazepam dose.

Equipment: Rota rod apparatus

PROCEDURE

1. Once the animals are weighed, number them.
2. Activate the device and choose a suitable speed (20–25 rpm).
3. Arrange the animals on the revolving rod one by one. More than one mouse may be placed. Record the moment at which the mouse drops from the revolving rod. A typical mouse usually falls off in three to five minutes.
4. Give all animals diazepam injections. Repeat step 3 trials after 30 minutes. Take note of the cutoff time.
5. Examine the animals' fall-off times both before and after receiving diazepam.

OBSERVATION

Dose of Diazepam: 4 mg/kg

The dose of **4 mg/kg of Diazepam** is used in murine studies to evaluate its **skeletal muscle relaxant properties** [2], because it helps achieve a balance between efficacy and safety. Diazepam, a benzodiazepine, exerts its muscle relaxant effects by enhancing the action of GABA (gamma-aminobutyric acid), which is an inhibitory neurotransmitter in the central nervous system1. This action results in decreased muscle tone and relaxation.

Table 5. Effect of Drug Treatment on Fall Time in Mice Following Dose Administration Based on Body Weight.

S. No.	Body weight (g)	Dose to be administered (mg)	Fall time (seconds)		% decrease in fall time
			Basel (A)	Treatment (B)	
1.	25	0.1	60	45	25.00%
2.	30	0.12	58	42	31.03%
3.	32	0.128	62	43	30.65%
4.	35	0.14	63	42	34.38%
5.	33	0.132	64	44	30.16%

% decrease= A-BA×100. This formula isusedto calculate the percentage decrease in fall time. Table **5** is followed by the reference [3].

INFERENCE

As the locomotor activity score decreased in rats given chlorpromazine, it was discovered that the drug had CNS depressive properties.

CONCLUSION

The experiment successfully demonstrated that skeletal muscle relaxants, such as diazepam and baclofen, dramatically impacted the motor coordination and balance of mice. This was demonstrated by a reduction in the amount of time that the rodents spent on the

revolving rod. It was discovered that the Rotarod apparatus is both dependable and sensitive for assessing the effects of skeletal muscle relaxants, which in turn provides significant information regarding the pharmacodynamics of these substances. The purpose of this test is to investigate the processes that are responsible for the activity of possible muscle relaxants and to screen new medicines. The findings have significant repercussions for the creation of therapeutic drugs for illnesses that need muscular relaxation, such as spasticity or muscle spasms, while also taking into consideration the potential adverse effects that are associated with motor coordination.

REFERENCES

[1]   Standaert DG, Young AB. Treatment of central nervous system degenerative disorders. Goodman & Gilaman's The Pharmacological Basis of Therapeutics 2006; pp. 527-45.

[2]   Goodman LS, Gilman A. The pharmacological basis of therapeutics. Macmillan New York. 1970.

[3]   Veena NS, Sivaji K, Benerji GV, Babu MF, Kumari DR. Skeletal muscle relaxant property of diazepam by using rotarod on albino mice. Indian J Basic Appl Med Res 2015; 4(4): 714-21.

CHAPTER 11

Effect of Drugs on the Locomotor Activity of Mice using Actophotometer

OBJECTIVE

To study the effect of drugs on the locomotor activity of mice using an actophotometer.

PRINCIPLE

The majority of medications that affect the central nervous system have an impact on how humans and animals move. Alcohol and other CNS depressants, like barbiturates, lower motor activity, whereas stimulants, like amphetamines and caffeine, boost it. Stated differently, locomotor activity can be indexed as ameasure of mental activity during waking hours. An actophotometer is a simple tool to use to monitor locomotor activity. It uses photoelectric cells that are wired into a circuit with a counter to function. When the light from the animal stops the light from landing on the photocell, a count is made. Actophotometers may have an arena in which the animal moves that can be square or circular. Rats and mice can both be employed in tests [1].

REQUIREMENT

Animal: Mice weighing 20-25 grams

Drugs: Chlorpromazine hydrochloride

Equipment: Actophotometer

PROCEDURE

1. Weigh each animal and assign a number.
2. After turning on the apparatus, put each mouse in the activity cage for ten minutes at a time. Each animal's basal activity score should be noted.
3. After 30 minutes of chlorpromazine injection, retest each mouse for activity scores for ten minutes. Observe how the activity changes before and after the administration of chlorpromazine.
4. Determine the motor activity drop as a percentage. % decrease= A-BA×100

Table 6. The effect of diazepam on locomotor activity in mice: evaluation of dose-dependent cns depression.

S. No.	Body Weight	Dose to be Administered	Basel (A)	Treatment (B)	Difference (A-B)	% Decrease in Locomotor Activity
1.	25	0.075	120	70	50	41.67%
2.	30	0.09	13	65	65	50.00%
3.	32	0.096	125	60	65	52.00%
4.	35	0.105	135	55	80	59.26%
5.	34	0.103	140	58	82	58.57%
6.	33	0.099	128	62	66	51.56%

Dose of chlorpromazine: 3mg/kg. Table **6** is followed by reference [2].

INFERENCE

As the locomotor activity score decreased in rats given chlorpromazine, it was discovered that the drug had CNS depressive properties [3].

CONCLUSION

The research effectively revealed that the central nervous system stimulants like caffeine and amphetamines enhanced locomotor activity in mice, whilst the central nervous system depressant diazepam decreased movement. This finding aligns with the pharmacological effects known to be associated with these substances. The actophotometer was a significant instrument for preclinical screening of medications that could potentially affect motor functions, as it provided a dependable and effective method for monitoring changes in locomotor activity [4]. Not only do these findings confirm the use of this method in evaluating the behavioral effects of medications, but they also highlight the significance of this method in an effort to comprehend the pharmacodynamics of substances that are active in the central nervous system. The findings have wider-ranging implications for the development of drugs, particularly for compounds that are intended to treat neurological or psychiatric diseases, which are conditions in which the modulation of motor activity is highly important.

REFERENCES

[1]   Patel C, Patel R, Kesharwani A, Rao L, Jain NS. Central cholinergic transmission modulates endocannabinoid-induced marble-burying behavior in mice. Behav Brain Res 2025; 476: 115252. [http://dx.doi.org/10.1016/j.bbr.2024.115252] [PMID: 39278464]

[2]   Simón VM, Parra A, Miñarro J, Arenas MC, Vinader-Caerols C, Aguilar MA. Predicting how equipotent doses of chlorpromazine, haloperidol, sulpiride, raclopride and clozapine reduce locomotor

activity in mice. Eur Neuropsychopharmacol 2000; 10(3): 159-64.
[http://dx.doi.org/10.1016/S0924-977X(00)00070-5] [PMID: 10793317]

[3]   Messiha FS. Anti-depressant action of caesium chloride and its modification of chlorpromazine toxicity in mice. Br J Pharmacol 1978; 64(1): 9-12.
[http://dx.doi.org/10.1111/j.1476-5381.1978.tb08634.x] [PMID: 698485]

[4]   López-Muñoz F, Alamo C. cuenca E., Shen W. W., Clervoy P., Rubio G. History of the discovery and clinical introduction of chlorpromazine. Ann Clin Psychiatry 2005; 17(3): 113-35.
[http://dx.doi.org/10.1080/10401230591002002] [PMID: 16433053]

CHAPTER 12

Anticonvulsant Effect of Drugs by MES & PTZ Method

OBJECTIVE

To study the anticonvulsant effect of drugs by the MES & PTZ method.

Epilepsy

Epilepsy is a chronic neurological disorder characterized by recurrent seizures, which are sudden and abnormal bursts of electrical activity in the brain. These seizures can vary in type, intensity, and frequency and may result in alterations in behavior, sensation, or consciousness.

Pathophysiology of Epilepsy

Seizures occur due to an imbalance between excitatory and inhibitory neurotransmission in the brain:

1. **Hyperexcitability:** Excessive firing of excitatory neurons due to enhanced activity of glutamate or reduced inhibition by GABA.
2. **Hypersynchrony:** Groups of neurons fire in a highly synchronized manner, leading to abnormal electrical discharges.
3. **Structural or Metabolic Alterations:** Changes in ion channels, neurotransmitter levels, or neuronal circuitry predisposed to seizures.

Types of Epileptic Seizures

The International League Against Epilepsy (ILAE) classifies seizures into two major types:

1. Focal (Partial) Seizures
   ○ Originate in a specific area of one hemisphere of the brain.
   ○ **Simple Focal Seizures:** No loss of consciousness; symptoms depend on the affected brain area (*e.g.*, motor, sensory).

- **Complex Focal Seizures:** Impaired awareness may be accompanied by automatisms (*e.g.*, lip-smacking).

2. Generalized Seizures

- Involve both hemispheres from the onset.
- **Tonic-Clonic (Grand Mal) Seizures:** Characterized by stiffening (tonic phase) followed by jerking movements (clonic phase).
- **Absence (Petit Mal) Seizures:** Brief episodes of staring or loss of awareness.
- **Myoclonic Seizures:** Sudden, brief muscle jerks.
- **Atonic Seizures:** Sudden loss of muscle tone, causing falls.
- **Tonic Seizures:** Sustained muscle contractions.
- **Clonic Seizures:** Rhythmic jerking movements.

Diagnosis of Epilepsy

1. Clinical History
   - Detailed account of seizure events, including triggers, duration, and associated symptoms.
   - Family and medical history.
2. Electroencephalogram (EEG)
   - Records electrical activity in the brain to detect abnormal patterns associated with epilepsy.
   - Interictal spikes or sharp waves suggest epilepsy.
3. Neuroimaging
   - **MRI:** To identify structural abnormalities (*e.g.*, tumors, cortical dysplasia).
   - **CT Scan:** Used in emergencies to detect acute lesions.
4. Blood Tests
   - Identify metabolic or infectious causes.
5. Genetic Testing
   - Performed in cases of suspected genetic epilepsies

PRINCIPLE

In experimental animals, epilepsy of various types, including grand mal, petit mal, and psychomotor type, can be investigated. Anticonvulsant medications are tested in laboratory animals using two ways to examine convulsion: chemo-convulsion caused by pentylenetetrazol, which causes clonic type convulsion in humans, and Maximum Electroshock (MES) generated convulsions in animals that simulate grandmal epilepsy [1]. Convulsion electroshock is administered *via* the ocular electrodes in MES. Cortical excitation is created through ocular stimulation [2]. The MES convulsion occurs in five stages.

1. Tonic flexion
2. Tonic extensor
3. Clonic convulsion
4. Stupor
5. Recovery/death

It is advised that students have a solid understanding of the pharmacology of anti-epileptic drugs before carrying out this experiment. A substance is deemed to have anti-convulsant qualities if it lowers or eliminates the extensor phase of MES convulsions in both rats and mice.

REQUIREMENT

Animal: Rats weighing between 150 and 200 grams.

Drugs: Make a stock solution and administer 25 mg/kg of phenytoin.

Equipment: An electroconvulsimeter, a cornel electrode (150 mA current for 0.2 sec), and a stopwatch.

PROCEDURE

1. Weigh and number the animals. Divide them into two groups, each with four or five rats. One group receives drug treatment, while the other serves as the control.
2. Hold the animals securely, and then apply the recommended current while placing corneal electrodes on the cornea. Observe the various convulsion stages.
3. Replicate with additional members of the control group.
4. Inject a batch of four to five rats with phenytoin I.P. After 30 minutes, the animals were made to undergo electroconvulsions.
5. MES convulsions show a reduction in duration or elimination of the tonic extensor [3].

Table 7. Observation of seizure phases and recovery in rodents following seizure induction.

S. No.	Onset time (sec)	Tonic limb flexor (sec)	Tonic extensor (sec)	clonus (sec)	Stupor (sec)	Recovery (sec)	Non-Extensor Seizure
1.	35	5	10	20	60	120	Yes
2.	40	6	12	18	55	115	No
3.	38	7	11	22	62	130	Yes
4.	42	5	13	19	58	125	No

(Table 7) cont.....

S. No.	Onset time (sec)	Tonic limb flexor (sec)	Tonic extensor (sec)	clonus (sec)	Stupor (sec)	Recovery (sec)	Non-Extensor Seizure
5.	37	6	10	21	61	128	Yes

Dose: Phenytoin 25mg/kg. Table **7** is followed by the reference [4].

INFERENCE

The medication's ability to reduce or eliminate the tonic-extensor phase is regarded as an anticonvulsant feature. Phenytoin eliminates tonic-extensors generated by MES.

REPORT

The effect of the anticonvulsant drug is observed by the application of the MES and PTZ method.

CONCLUSION

All three medications- phenytoin, valproate, and diazepam- were observed to successfully demonstrate their anticonvulsant effects in the MES and PTZ seizure models through the laboratory experiment. In the MES model, phenytoin and valproate were successful in suppressing tonic-clonic seizures. On the other hand, diazepam showed substantial efficacy in preventing generalized seizures in the PTZ model. The findings of this study provide further evidence that these medications play a role in regulating brain activity and preventing seizures. The research highlights the significance of the MES and PTZ procedures as reliable instruments for preclinical anticonvulsant screening. The significance of these models in the process of developing medications for epilepsy and other neurological problems is brought to light by these findings, which provide credence to the clinical application of pharmaceuticals that were tested for the management of a variety of seizure disorders.

REFERENCES

[1]   Snehunsu A, Mukunda N, Satish Kumar MC, *et al.* Evaluation of anti-epileptic property of *Marsilea quadrifolia* Linn. in maximal electroshock and pentylenetetrazole-induced rat models of epilepsy. Brain Inj 2013; 27(13-14): 1707-14.
[http://dx.doi.org/10.3109/02699052.2013.831121] [PMID: 24215095]

[2]   Nsour WM, Lau CBS, Wong ICK. Review on phytotherapy in epilepsy. Seizure 2000; 9(2): 96-107.
[http://dx.doi.org/10.1053/seiz.1999.0378] [PMID: 10845732]

[3]   Gastaut H, Roger J, Ocjahchi S, Ttmsit M, Broughton R. An electro-clinical study of generalized epileptic seizures of tonic expression. Epilepsia 1963; 4(1-4): 15-44.
[http://dx.doi.org/10.1111/j.1528-1157.1963.tb05206.x] [PMID: 13963212]

[4]   Leite JP, Bortolotto ZA, Cavalheiro EA. Spontaneous recurrent seizures in rats: An experimental model of partial epilepsy. Neurosci Biobehav Rev 1990; 14(4): 511-7.
[http://dx.doi.org/10.1016/S0149-7634(05)80076-4] [PMID: 2287490]

CHAPTER 13

Drugs Used for Anti-Cationic Activity and Stereotype-Like Behavior in Murinea

OBJECTIVES

1. To study drug (phenothiazines) induced catatonia (extrapyramidal side effect in rats).
2. To study the anticatatonic (antiparkinsonian) effect of scopolamine.

PRINCIPLE

It is known that antipsychotic medications of the phenothiazine and butyrophenone types cause extrapyramidal adverse effects in humans. These side effects, which include tremors, rigidity, and akinesia, are referred to as Parkinson-like since one of the main clinical symptoms of Parkinson's disease is difficulty moving. The side effects of antipsychotic medication are brought on by excessive blocking of the extrapyramidal motor system's dopamine receptors. Consequently, phenothiazines (perphenazine or chlorpromazine) are frequently used to cause extrapyramidal symptoms similar to Parkinson's symptoms in lab animals and to research medications that treat Parkinson's disease. Students are recommended to be familiar with the pharmacology of anti-Parkinsonian medications before conducting this experiment [1, 2].

REQUIREMENTS

Animal: Rats (150-200 g)

Drugs:

- Perphenazine (dose: 5 mg/kg i.p.; make a stock solution with 1 mg/ml of the medication, and then inject 0.5 ml per 100 g of the animal's body weight).
- Scopolamine (dosage: 2 mg/kg; inject 0.5 ml/100 g of the animal's body weight after making a stock solution containing 0.4 mg/ml of the medication). Equipment: Two wooden blocks, one measuring three centimeters in height and the other measuring nine centimeters.

Cationic Activity of Drugs

Cationic activity refers to the ability of drugs to carry a positive charge and interact with negatively charged biological molecules or structures such as cell membranes, DNA, RNA, or proteins. This property is particularly important in certain drug classes, as it significantly influences their mechanism of action, pharmacodynamics, and therapeutic applications.

Mechanism of Cationic Activity

Drugs with cationic properties interact with negatively charged components through electrostatic interactions. For example:

1. **Cell Membranes**: Many bacterial membranes have a negative charge due to phospholipids and lipopolysaccharides. Cationic drugs bind to these sites, disrupting membrane integrity, leading to cell lysis or altered permeability.
2. **Nucleic Acids**: Some cationic drugs interact with negatively charged DNA or RNA, inhibiting replication, transcription, or translation.
3. **Protein Targets**: Cationic drugs may also bind to negatively charged functional groups on enzymes or structural proteins, affecting their activity.

Examples of Drugs with Cationic Activity

1. **Aminoglycosides**:

• Bind to the negatively charged 16S ribosomal RNA in the bacterial 30S subunit, disrupting protein synthesis.

2. **Quaternary Ammonium Compounds**:

• Act as disinfectants by disrupting bacterial and fungal cell membranes.

3. **Antimalarial Drugs (*e.g.*, Chloroquine)**:

• Bind to negatively charged heme in the parasite's food vacuole, preventing detoxification and leading to parasite death.

4. **Polymyxins (*e.g.*, Polymyxin B, Colistin)**:

• Interact with the negatively charged phosphate groups in the bacterial outer membrane, disrupting its structure and function.

Significance of Cationic Activity

• **Antimicrobial Action**: Many antibiotics and antiseptics rely on cationic activity

to target pathogens selectively.
- **Target Specificity**: The electrostatic interactions enhance the drug's ability to selectively bind to microbial or diseased tissues.
- **Drug Delivery**: Cationic nanoparticles or liposomes are used to enhance drug delivery by interacting with negatively charged cell surfaces or DNA.

PROCEDURE

1. Weigh and number the animal. Divide the animals into two groups: one for studying the scopolamine effect and another for assessing the perphenazine impact (control group). Each group should contain a minimum of five animals (Tables **10** & **11**).
2. Use perphenazine injections to manage animals. Note the catatonic response's severity.
3. After taking perphenazine, note the degree of catatonia at 5, 15, 30, 45, 60, 90, and 120 minutes.
4. The animals in the second group were given scopolamine injections, followed by a 30-minute injection of perphenazine. Assess the degree of catatonia by observing and scoring as in step 2.
5. Examine the difference in the two groups' catatonic responses' beginning and intensity. Draw a graph with time plotted on the x-axis. Keep in mind that there were differences in the onset and intensity of catatonic reactions in both groups [3 - 6].

Table 10. Effect of Perphenazine (5 mg/kg, I.P) on Catatonia Induction in Mice at Different Time Intervals.

S. No.	Weight of Animal	Dose	Dose to be Administered	Mean Catatonia After Minutes of PERP Treatment					
			Perphenazine (mg)	15	30	45	60	90	120
1.	180	Perphenazine (5mg/kg)	0.9	0.5	1.0	2.5	3.5	3.0	1.5
2.	185		0.92	0.5	1.5	2.8	3.8	3.2	1.8
3.	205		1.02	0.8	1.2	3.0	4.0	3.3	1.7
4.	210		1.05	0.7	1.4	2.9	4.2	3.5	1.6
5.	200		1	0.6	1.3	2.7	3.9	3.1	1.5
	Mean		0.798	0.62	1.28	2.78	3.8	3.2	1.6

Table 11. Effect of Scopolamine (2 mg/kg, I.P) Pretreatment on Perphenazine (5 mg/kg, I.P)-Induced Catatonia in Mice at Different Time Intervals.

S. No	Weight of Animal	Dose	Dose to be Administered		Mean Catatonia After Minutes of PERP Treatment					
			Scopolamine (mg)	Perphenazine (mg)	15	30	45	60	90	120
1.	180	Scopolamine (2mg/kg)+ Perphenazine (5mg/kg)	0.36	0.90	0.0	0.5	1.0	1.8	1.5	0.8
2.	190		0.38	0.95	0.2	0.7	1.1	2.0	1.7	0.9
3.	200		0.40	1.00	0.1	0.6	1.2	1.9	1.6	0.7
4.	205		0.41	1.025	0.2	0.8	1.3	2.1	1.8	1.0
5.	195		0.39	0.975	0.1	0.6	1.1	1.8	1.5	0.9
	Mean		**0.388**	**0.97**	**0.12**	**0.64**	**1.14**	**1.92**	**1.62**	**0.86**

INFERENCE: Scopolamine has an anti-catatonic effect by lowering the mean catatonic score.

CONCLUSION

Through the use of mouse models, the experiment successfully illustrates the opposing effects of dopaminergic agonists and antagonists on stereotypy and catatonia. The function that dopaminergic stimulants play in boosting dopamine activity is highlighted by the fact that they can cause stereotypical behaviors to rise. However, dopamine antagonists such as haloperidol inhibited dopaminergic pathways, which resulted in the induction of catatonic states. This was the opposite of what was expected. Levodopa was able to successfully reverse catatonia, demonstrating that it has the potential to be used as a treatment agent in illnesses that involve motor dysfunction, such as Parkinson's disease. Based on these findings, the utilization of rat models for the purpose of researching the dopaminergic modulation of motor control and screening medications for extrapyramidal illnesses is considered valid. It is essential to have such models in order to discover therapeutic drugs that can restore motor function while simultaneously limiting adverse effects.

REFERENCES

[1]   Irwin S. Comprehensive observational assessment: Ia. A systematic, quantitative procedure for assessing the behavioral and physiologic state of the mouse. Psychopharmacology (Berl) 1968; 13(3): 222-57.
[http://dx.doi.org/10.1007/BF00401402] [PMID: 5679627]

[2]   Frank LA, Contri RV, Beck RCR, Pohlmann AR, Guterres SS. Improving drug biological effects by encapsulation into polymeric nanocapsules. Wiley Interdiscip Rev Nanomed Nanobiotechnol 2015; 7(5): 623-39.

[http://dx.doi.org/10.1002/wnan.1334] [PMID: 25641603]

[3]   Klawans HL Jr, Rubovits R, Patel BC, Weiner WJ. Cholinergic and anticholinergic influences on amphetamine-induced stereotyped behavior. J Neurol Sci 1972; 17(3): 303-8.
[http://dx.doi.org/10.1016/0022-510X(72)90035-4] [PMID: 4653965]

[4]   Thippeswamy BS, Mishra B, Veerapur VP, Gupta G. Anxiolytic activity of Nymphaea alba Linn. in mice as experimental models of anxiety. Indian J Pharmacol 2011; 43(1): 50-5.
[http://dx.doi.org/10.4103/0253-7613.75670] [PMID: 21455422]

[5]   Duty S, Jenner P. Animal models of Parkinson's disease: a source of novel treatments and clues to the cause of the disease. Br J Pharmacol 2011; 164(4): 1357-91.
[http://dx.doi.org/10.1111/j.1476-5381.2011.01426.x] [PMID: 21486284]

[6]   Crawley JN. Exploratory behavior models of anxiety in mice. Neurosci Biobehav Rev 1985; 9(1): 37-44.
[http://dx.doi.org/10.1016/0149-7634(85)90030-2] [PMID: 2858080]

CHAPTER 14

Study of Anxiolytic Activity of Drugs Using the Murine

OBJECTIVE

To studies the Anxiolytic Activity of Drugs Using Murines.

Anxiety

Anxiety is a natural response to perceived threats. It involves a heightened state of alertness that is accompanied by physiological changes, such as an increased heart rate and muscle tension. This response, often referred to as the "fight or flight" mechanism, has evolutionary roots and is meant to help individuals deal with danger.

However, modern stressors, such as work pressure, financial difficulties, or personal relationships, can trigger this response unnecessarily, leading to chronic anxiety in some individuals [1].

Symptoms of Anxiety
Emotional Symptoms

1. Excessive worry or fear.
2. Feelings of restlessness or being "on edge."
3. Irritability or frustration.
4. A sense of impending doom or danger.

Physical Symptoms

1. Rapid heartbeat (tachycardia).
2. Shortness of breath or hyperventilation.
3. Sweating or chills.
4. Trembling or shaking.
5. Muscle tension or fatigue.
6. Nausea, dizziness, or gastrointestinal disturbances.
7. Difficulty sleeping (insomnia).

Cognitive Symptoms

1. Trouble concentrating or staying focused.
2. Overthinking or racing thoughts.
3. Catastrophizing (assuming the worst will happen).
4. Indecisiveness or feeling overwhelmed.

Causes of Anxiety

Biological Factors

1. **Neurotransmitter Imbalance**: Abnormal levels of serotonin, dopamine, and Gamma-Aminobutyric Acid (GABA) can contribute to anxiety.
2. **Genetics**: A family history of anxiety disorders increases the risk.
3. **Brain Structure**: Hyperactivity in the amygdala, which processes fear, may play a role.

Psychological Factors

1. **Past Trauma**: Experiencing traumatic events can increase susceptibility to anxiety.
2. **Learned Behavior**: Growing up in an environment of fear or excessive worry may predispose individuals to anxiety.

Environmental Factors

1. **Stressful Life Events**: Financial difficulties, relationship problems, or academic pressures.
2. **Substance Abuse**: Alcohol, caffeine, or drugs can exacerbate anxiety.
3. **Chronic Illness**: Conditions like diabetes, cardiovascular disease, or chronic pain can contribute to anxiety.

Types of Anxiety Disorders

1. Generalized Anxiety Disorder (GAD):

- Persistent and excessive worry about everyday matters.
- Symptoms last for at least six months.

2. Panic Disorder:

- Characterized by sudden and intense episodes of fear (panic attacks).
- Symptoms include chest pain, palpitations, and feelings of losing control.

3. Social Anxiety Disorder (SAD):

• Intense fear of being judged or embarrassed in social situations.
• Can lead to avoidance of social interactions.

4. Specific Phobias:

• Extreme fear of a particular object or situation (*e.g.*, heights, spiders).
• The fear is disproportionate to the actual danger.

5. Obsessive-Compulsive Disorder (OCD):

• Characterized by intrusive thoughts (obsessions) and repetitive behaviors (compulsions).

6. Post-Traumatic Stress Disorder (PTSD):

• Develops after exposure to a traumatic event.
• Symptoms include flashbacks, nightmares, and heightened arousal.

7. Separation Anxiety Disorder:

• Fear of being separated from attachment figures, more common in childrenmbut can affect adults.

PRINCIPLE

Anxiety is characterized as a state of unease, ambiguity, and strain resulting from the expectation of a perceived or hypothetical danger. The elevated zero-maze test is a behavioral anxiety test that uses rats' naturalistic avoidance behavior as its basis in places that are open and lofty. It resembles the elevated plus maze, which is more popular, and the closed arms are positioned in a circle, removing the middle portion, which eliminates the unclear interpretation of the amount of time spent in the traditional central square style. An elevated (40-centimeter) white or black circular maze with an inner diameter of 30 cm and an outside diameter of 45 cm is what it looks like. The mouse can explore a 6 cm wide runway ring that is separated into four quadrants, with two "open" wall-free quadrants and two "closed" quadrants with walls that are 12 cm high. A 2-3 mm ridge surrounds the open quadrants to keep mice from falling off the walls. The thickness is 0.75 cm [2].

REQUIREMENTS

Animal: Mice

Drugs: Diazepam

Equipment: Zero-maze

PROCEDURE

1. Number and weigh the animals, and split them into two groups, with a minimum of six mice in each. One group receives drug treatment while the other serves as the control.

2. Each animal should be placed with its back to the closed arm in the open arm. Set the stopwatch to begin, and throughout the next six minutes, record the following parameters.
    a. Latency to enter to open arm
    b. Average time each animal spends in the open/ closed arm.
    c. Total number of entries in the open arm
    d. Stretchings

3. After every attempt, wipe the maze down using tissue paper.

4. After 30 minutes, inject the test group with diazepam; then, treat each animal as previously said, making note of all the parameters as in step 2.

Observation Table **12** is given below and the table is followed by reference [3].

REPORT: The anxiolytic effects of drugs are investigated in mice and rats.

Table 12. Assessment of Anxiolytic Activity of Diazepam in Mice Using the Elevated Zero Maze Model.

S. No.	Group	Animal Weight (g)	Dose (mg/kg)	Time in Open Quadrant (sec)	Time in Closed Quadrant (sec)	No. of Open Entries
1	Control	25	0	40	260	2
2	Diazepam (1 mg/kg)	25.5	1	85	215	5
3	Diazepam (2 mg/kg)	26	2	125	175	7
	Mean			83.33	216.66	4.66

CONCLUSION

The study aimed to evaluate the anxiolytic activity of drugs using standard behavioral models in mice and rats. Animal models like the Elevated Plus Maze

(EPM) and Open Field Test (OFT) were employed to assess anxiety-related behaviors. Test drugs, including benzodiazepines like diazepam, were compared against control groups to determine their efficacy in reducing anxiety. Behavioral parameters such as time spent in open arms (EPM) and central zone activity (OFT) were recorded. Diazepam significantly increased the exploration of open arms and central zones, indicating a reduction in anxiety levels. The findings validate these animal models as reliable tools for screening anxiolytic drugs and demonstrate the efficacy of diazepam as a standard anxiolytic agent. This study contributes to understanding the pharmacological basis of anxiety and aids in the development of novel therapeutic agents.

REFERENCES

[1]   Kilfoil T, Michel A, Montgomery D, Whiting RL. Effects of anxiolytic and anxiogenic drugs on exploratory activity in a simple model of anxiety in mice. Neuropharmacology 1989; 28(9): 901-5.
        [http://dx.doi.org/10.1016/0028-3908(89)90188-3] [PMID: 2572995]

[2]   Peng WH, Wu CR, Chen CS, Chen CF, Leu ZC, Hsieh MT. Anxiolytic effect of berberine on exploratory activity of the mouse in two experimental anxiety models: Interaction with drugs acting at 5-HT receptors. Life Sci 2004; 75(20): 2451-62.
        [http://dx.doi.org/10.1016/j.lfs.2004.04.032] [PMID: 15350820]

[3]   Shepherd JK, Grewal SS, Fletcher A, Bill DJ, Dourish CT. Behavioural and pharmacological characterisation of the elevated "zero-maze" as an animal model of anxiety. Psychopharmacology (Berl) 1994; 116(1): 56-64.
        [http://dx.doi.org/10.1007/BF02244871] [PMID: 7862931]

CHAPTER 15

Study of Local Anaesthetics by Different Methods

OBJECTIVE

To study the effect of local anesthetics by different methods.

PRINCIPLE

Local anesthetics impede impulse conduction *via* excitable membranes and nerve axons in a reversible manner. They act to inhibit pain perception and to create local or regional anesthesia. It is simple to study the local anesthetic property by employing any of the **3 *below mentioned*** techniques, namely; (a) nerve block anesthesia (Solman method), where the medication is administered in proximity to the nerve trunk; (b) surface anesthesia, where the medication is injected into the eye's conjunctiva and corneal reflux is observed toward a pointed object and (c) anesthesia infiltration (in which the medication is injected intradermally and the location is examined for pinprick sensitivity).

Local Anesthetics

Local anesthetics [1] are a class of drugs that temporarily block the transmission of nerve impulses, leading to a reversible loss of sensation in a specific area of the body. Unlike general anesthetics, local anesthetics do not cause loss of consciousness. They are widely used in medical and dental procedures to manage pain and facilitate minor surgeries, diagnostic procedures, and other interventions.

Mechanism of Action

Local anesthetics work by inhibiting the conduction of electrical impulses in nerve fibers [2]. This is achieved by:

1. **Targeting Sodium Channels**:
   ○ Local anesthetics bind to voltage-gated sodium channels in the nerve membrane.
   ○ This binding inhibits the influx of sodium ions, which is essential for the depolarization phase of the action potential.
2. **Blocking Nerve Conduction**:
   ○ When sodium channels are blocked, the nerve cannot generate or propagatemaction potentials.
   ○ This prevents the brain from receiving pain signals from the affected area.

Types of Local Anesthetics [3]

Based on Chemical Structure

1. **Ester-linked Anesthetics**:
   ○ Shorter duration of action due to rapid metabolism by plasma esterases.
   ○ Examples: Procaine, Chloroprocaine, Benzocaine.
2. **Amide-linked Anesthetics**:
   ○ Longer duration of action and slower metabolism by liver enzymes.
   ○ Examples: Lidocaine, Bupivacaine, Ropivacaine, Mepivacaine.

Based on Duration of Action

1. **Short-Acting**:
   ○ Examples: Procaine, Chloroprocaine.
2. **Intermediate-Acting**:
   ○ Examples: Lidocaine, Mepivacaine.
3. **Long-Acting**:
   ○ Examples: Bupivacaine, Ropivacaine.

Clinical Uses

1. **Topical Anesthesia**:
   ○ Applied directly to mucous membranes or skin.
   ○ Examples: Benzocaine, Lidocaine (in creams, sprays, gels).
2. **Infiltration Anesthesia**:
   ○ Injected into tissues for minor surgical procedures or wound suturing.
   ○ Examples: Lidocaine, Procaine.
3. **Nerve Block Anesthesia**:
   ○ Injected near a specific nerve or nerve plexus to block sensation in a larger area.
   ○ Examples: Bupivacaine, Ropivacaine.

4. **Spinal Anesthesia**:
   ○ Injected into the subarachnoid space to anesthetize lower body regions.
   ○ Examples: Lidocaine, Tetracaine.
5. **Epidural Anesthesia**:
   ○ Injected into the epidural space, commonly used in childbirth and surgeries.
   ○ Examples: Bupivacaine, Ropivacaine.
6. **Intravenous Regional Anesthesia (Bier Block)**:
   ○ An anesthetic is injected into a vein of an extremity, often combined with a tourniquet.
   ○ Example: Lidocaine.

Adverse Effects

While local anesthetics are generally safe when used correctly, adverse effects may occur due to systemic absorption, overdose, or allergic reactions.

1. **Central Nervous System (CNS)**:
   ○ Early symptoms: Restlessness, dizziness, tinnitus, metallic taste.
   ○ Severe symptoms: Seizures, respiratory depression, or coma.
2. **Cardiovascular System**:
   ○ Bradycardia, hypotension, or arrhythmias.
   ○ Bupivacaine, in particular, is associated with cardiotoxicity.
3. **Allergic Reactions**:
   ○ More common with ester-linked anesthetics due to the formation of Para-Aminobenzoic Acid (PABA), a known allergen.
4. **Local Tissue Toxicity**:
   ○ Prolonged use can cause nerve damage or tissue necrosis.

Contraindications

1. **Severe liver disease**: Amide anesthetics are metabolized in the liver and may accumulate.
2. **Allergy to local anesthetics**: Particularly ester-linked anesthetics.
3. **Heart conditions**: Use with caution in patients with arrhythmias or severe bradycardia.

REQUIREMENTS

Animal: frog

Drug: Procaine hydrochloride stock solution (1%w/v), hydrochloric acid (0.1N)

PROCEDURE

1. With the use of a pithing needle, decapitate the frog weighing between 100 and 150 grams and damage the upper portion of its spinal cord.
2. Make a pouch out of the abdominal walls by cutting up the abdomen and removing all of the organs.
3. Open up the cavity to reveal the spinal nerves.
4. Set the frog on the frog board with two of its hind legs hanging loosely from the board. Another option is to use a board that is nailed vertically to keep the frog's hind legs free to dangle.
5. Dip the right hind leg into the 0.1N HCl solution in the beaker. Observe the leg's fast reflex withdrawal.
6. Rinse the submerged leg under running water or in a beaker filled with regular saline.
7. Repeat the same with another leg.
8. Ten milliliters of 1% w/v procaine hydrochloride should be added to the abdominal pouch. The sciatic nerve flex feels the drug's local anesthetic effects. Allow the medication five minutes to take effect.
9. Submerge the hind legs of the right and left leg sequentially in the acid-filled beaker as previously.
10. Take note of the delay in the legs' reflexive withdrawal.

INFERENCE

The frog experiences local anesthesia upon direct injection of procaine hydrochloride to the nerve trunk, resulting in the blockage of foot withdrawal reflexes.

REPORT

A variety of techniques were used to study the effects of local anesthetics.

CONCLUSION

Within the scope of this investigation, the effects of local anesthetics were successfully demonstrated by the utilization of infiltration, surface, and nerve block techniques. While lignocaine, which has a rapid start and a moderate duration, has been shown to be beneficial for procedures that are performed for a short period of time, bupivacaine, which has a delayed onset but a longer duration, is better suited for operations that require protracted anesthesia. The findings provide evidence that sodium channel blocking plays a role in the mechanism of anesthesia, highlighting the importance of selecting a suitable drug based on the specific requirements of the clinical setting. The pharmacological properties of local anesthetics can be accurately evaluated using these experimental methodologies, which contribute to the creation of novel medicines that have efficacy and safety profiles that have been optimized. The findings of this study highlight the clinical significance of local anesthetics in the management of pain and in the performance of minor surgical procedures.

REFERENCES

[1]   Rioja Garcia E. Local Anesthetics. Veterinary Anesthesia and Analgesia. Wiley 2015; pp. 332-54.
       [http://dx.doi.org/10.1002/9781119421375.ch17]

[2]   Šimurina T, Mraović B, Župčić M, Graf Župčić S, Vulin M. Local anesthetics and steroids: Contraindications and complications - Clinical update. Acta Clin Croat 2019; 58 (Suppl. 1): 53-61.
       [http://dx.doi.org/10.20471/acc.2019.58.s1.08] [PMID: 31741560]

[3]   Flecknell PA, Thomas AA. Comparative Anesthesia and Analgesia of Laboratory Animals. Veterinary Anesthesia and Analgesia. Wiley 2015; pp. 754-63.
       [http://dx.doi.org/10.1002/9781119421375.ch39]

SUBJECT INDEX

www.ingramcontent.com/pod-product-compliance
Lightning Source LLC
Chambersburg PA
CBHW041448210326
41599CB00004B/180